AMERICAN YOGA

BARNES
&NOBLE
BOOKS
NEW YORK

AMERICAN YOGA

BY CARRIE SCHNEIDER

Photographs by Andy Ryan

AMERICAN YOGA

Photographs © 2003 Andy Ryan, Boston, MA, with the exception of:
Page 14, top: Lilias Folan courtesy WCET-TV, Cincinnati, OH
Pages 16–17: ELIOT ELISOFON/Time-Life Pictures/Getty Images
Page 23: Richard Freeman photograph © 2003 Tim Benko, Boulder, CO
Pages 30–31: © Jeremy Horner/CORBIS
Page 113: Stephen Cope photograph © 2003 Adam Mastoon, Housatonic, MA
Page 197: © Ric Ergenbright/CORBIS
Page 199: Sanskrit alphabet, courtesy of Ananda Ashram, Monroe, NY

For information contact:
Silver Lining Books, 122 Fifth Avenue, New York, NY 10011
212 633-4000

Barnes & Noble and colophon are registered trademarks.

    Publisher: Barbara J. Morgan
      Design: Richard J. Berenson
               Berenson Design & Books, Ltd., New York, NY
   Production: Della R. Mancuso
               Mancuso Associates, Inc., North Salem, NY

Library of Congress Cataloging-in-Publication Data is available on request.

ISBN 0-7607-4558-7

Printed in England

First Printing

To all the wonderful teachers and students
who offer themselves to the practice

CONTENTS

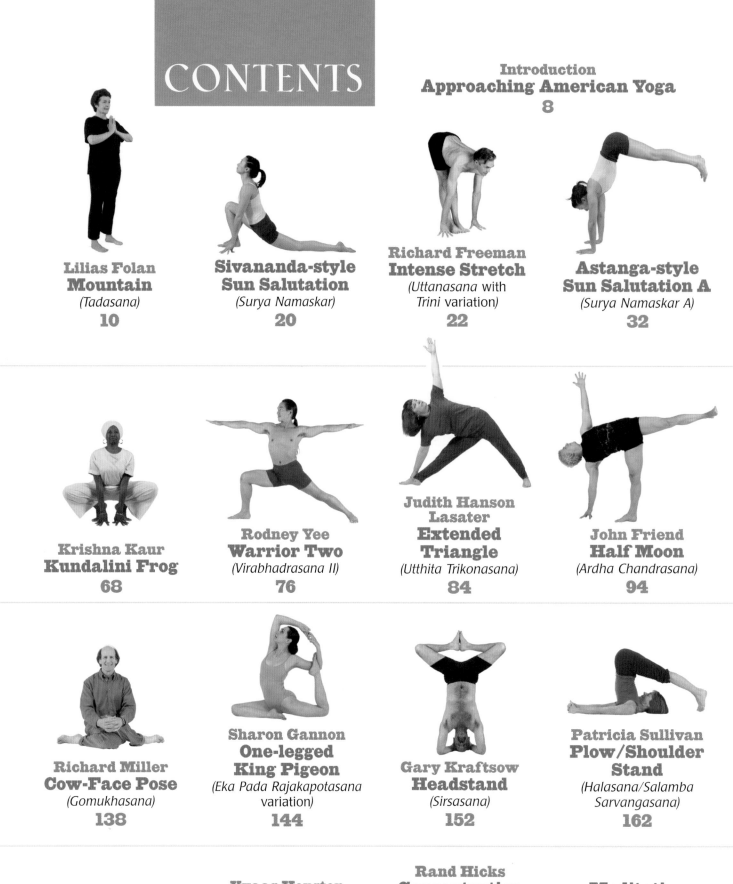

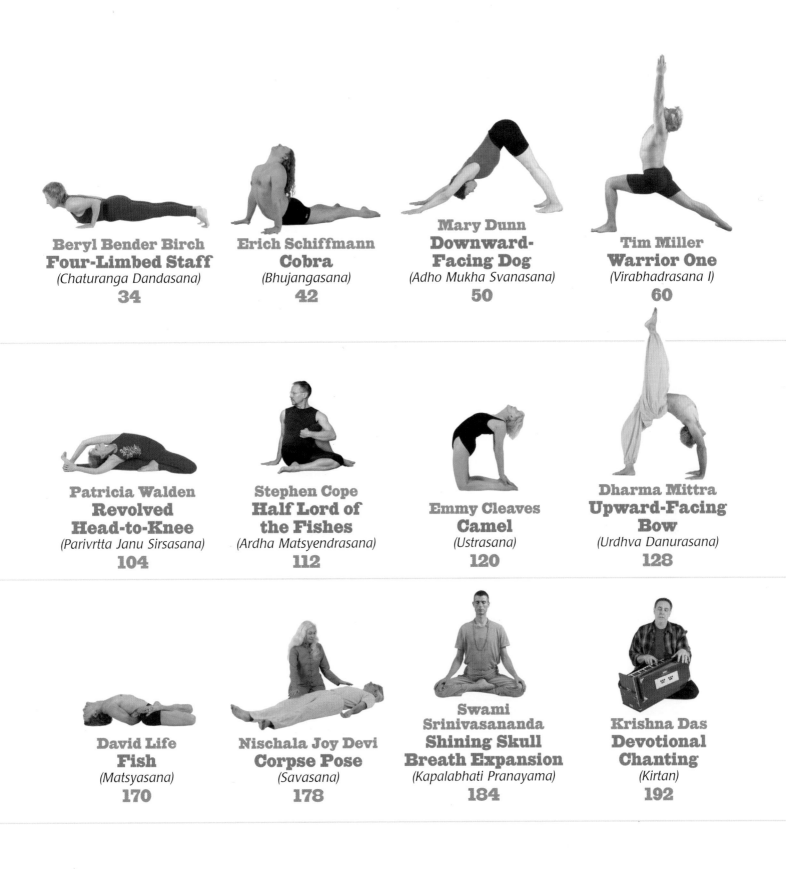

Introduction

APPROACHING AMERICAN YOGA

In October 1996, as a late-thirtysomething editor with a flagging interest in that career, I attended a conference at Kripalu Center for Yoga and Health, in Lenox, Massachusetts. The conference, directed by Stephen Cope—one of *American Yoga's* masters—showcased five styles of practice that kaleidoscoped into the concept for this book.

On Kripalu's second floor, in a room heated to 105 degrees, hard-bodied practitioners in bathing suits performed Bikram Yoga's twenty-six postures, two sets each, spurred on by the tough love of the Hollywood guru Emmy Cleaves. Next door, Lilias Folan transmitted the brand of sweet expansion with which she has plied TV audiences for more than a quarter century. In the auditorium, Beryl Bender Birch led the muscular ballet of Astanga Yoga, while a few doors down, men and women in loose cotton clothing moved through what Kripalu Yoga calls "meditation in motion." And one floor below it all, Iyengar Yoga teacher Judith Lasater worked the room—"Drop your hip and look up. Now you're doing Triangle, yes or no?"—asking her students to forget whatever they thought they knew.

In every one of those classes, what was being taught was American yoga.

As is its wont, this country has taken a tradition born on distant shores and changed it subtly with its embrace. Twenty million people now practice yoga nationwide, and the masters profiled here are excellent reasons for that. Their teachings invoke often radically different schools of yoga—some nearly acrobatic, some more contemplative and slow, and some that involve no postures, or asanas, at all. But whether they wear Lycra shorts or orange robes, these teachers help us yoke (*yug*, in Sanskrit) the power of the body and the mind toward liberation of the soul.

In reading the stories of how they came to the practice, you will find their paths as diverse as their approaches to teaching it. Major themes recur, however.

As ancient Sanskrit texts were to great Indian yoga masters for millennia, books were often the root teachers for these keen students. The books that drew them in varied. Those seekers with a propensity for knowledge or intellect were lured by translations of core literature like the Vedas and Upanishads. The more devotional among them were inspired by stories like Paramahansa Yogananda's *Autobiography of a Yogi.* But at first or eventually they all came upon a primer—*Light on Yoga* by B.K.S. Iyengar, Swami Satchidananda's *Integral Yoga Hatha,* or Swami Vishnu-devananda's *The Complete Illustrated Book of Yoga*—that paved their way in the practice of yoga..

Their paths also tended to be affected by the work of another writer, Aldous Huxley, whose 1954 book *The Doors of Perception* popularized a quicker route to expanding consciousness. Huxley noted that in the sixteenth century, Spaniards in the New World wrote that the Indians of Mexico and the American Southwest "venerated peyote as though it were a deity." By the late 1960s and early '70s, young Americans were engaged in similar homage. But the Indian yoga master Swami Satchidananda gently rerouted the hippies who flocked to study with him after he inaugurated the Woodstock Festival in 1969. "They said they wanted to expand their consciousness," he said in his biography, *Sri Swami Satchidananda: Apostle of Peace.* "But when the drugs failed them they turned to yoga consciousness. As they continued the purifying yoga practice, their use of drugs simply fell away naturally."

Whatever initiated their process of Self-discovery, the guidance of a guru or mentor played a major role in the progression of American yogis. These pages contain their recollections of the spiritual leader or leaders who shaped the journey, often illustrated by personal photographs that add texture to the tale. And through their own words and images, these longtime devotees now fulfill that function for a whole new generation of practitioners.

By observing these yoga masters in the postures they describe, you will come to understand at least one fundamental tenet of their teaching. Each master explains the wisdom or beauty of the asana—what I call the "yoga of the pose"—as well as how you might miss the pose and what you need to do to connect. Since not all the postures

Posture instruction throughout the book is generally shown and described on the right side of the body. Be sure to practice all single-side postures alternately, and remember to hold each asana for at least five slow, steady breaths.

pictured here may be appropriate for your personal practice, adaptations or variations are included to provide safe, functional alternatives that deliver their essence. The step-by-step instructions following each master's pose are culled from a conglomerate of traditions and may not necessarily reflect that master's teaching. For more of a particular teacher's wisdom, see the Resources section on page 208.

No matter which lineage they follow or style they teach, the men and women in these pages would say that their sights are set on the same *darshana,* or view. And that is none other than the goal of yoga: unfettered consciousness. The body is the temple of our soul, so we keep it pure and strong as a worthy vehicle for divinity. Yet the practice of yoga, here as in time immemorial, is to realize that we are something more than the body and the mind.

Whether you are a seasoned practitioner or new to the practice, *American Yoga* is written for you. We begin where we are, these great teachers will tell you. Their instruction will show you how to do yoga; their example will help you be it.

Carrie Schneider
August 2003

Lilias Folan

Mountain
(Tadasana)

"And now begins yoga," a voice inside Lilias Folan proclaims when she presses her palms together and stands at the ready in Mountain pose. The tenor of that voice is strong and sweet and clear. But there was a time in her life when Lilias could no longer hear it.

In 1964, twenty-eight years old and five years into her marriage, Lilias went to her doctor with what she calls a litany of complaints. From the outside it looked as if she was living the American dream, complete with a loving husband, two children, a golden retriever, and a four-bedroom house in the well-heeled community of Darien, Connecticut. But all was not well, and maintaining the pretense that everything was had become exhausting. Lilias told her physician that her back ached from lifting her baby boys. She admitted she was smoking too much, and she complained that her energy level lagged notably by midday. But there was one more thing she was reluctant to talk about—the "gloom cloud" that had hung over her for as long as she could remember.

As a child born to children, as she phrases it, Lilias had known great unhappiness before and after the pain of her parents' difficult divorce. The way she got through it all was by communing with a force within her heart she thought of as her "friend," a warm, unnameable presence that countered the turmoil she was undergoing at home. As her situation eased a bit, Lilias forgot about that inner wellspring of strength and peace—until she had cause to seek it out again in her late teens. But when she reached inside, she came up empty. It seemed her friend was gone. And even the joy she came to know when she had her own young family did not make up for the loss.

Lilias had hoped that her doctor would write her a prescription for the little yellow pills other Darien housewives were gobbling down like M&Ms. Instead, he recommended a program of physical exercise. As chance had it, Lilias had just read a book called *Yoga, Youth and Reincarnation.* So she decided to forgo the popular options of tennis and golf to attend a hatha yoga class at her local YWCA.

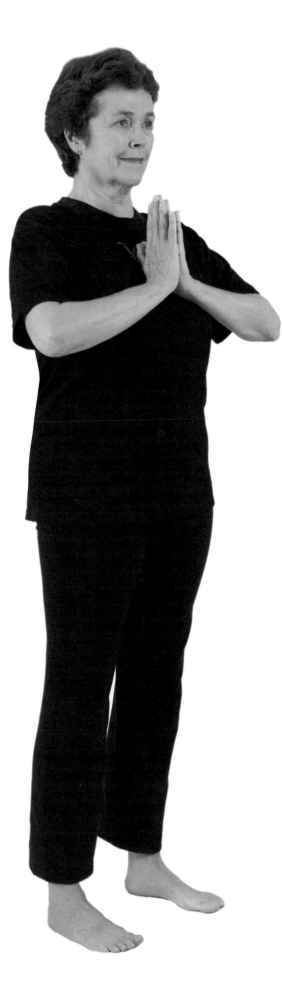

Beyond serious soreness in muscles she hadn't known she had, the experience engendered a sense of wonder and exploration that drew her back to class again and again.

The instructor at the Y taught Lilias the basics of yoga asanas, or postures, but often skipped the all-important final relaxation known as Corpse pose, which Lilias had instantly perceived to be key. Primed to explore yoga's deeper purpose, she began hopping the train to New York City, which at that time was "just bustling with it," she recalls. "India was coming to you; you didn't have to go to India."

At the Sivananda Yoga Center she studied with its founder, Swami Vishnu-devananda (p. 187), whom she describes as "brisk, inspired, and inspiring." She found classes with him to be "a hoot—this wonderfully round man who didn't look like he had muscles at all but could put his feet behind his head," she says. She also encountered Swami Satchidananda (p. 178), who had been a popular figure since he inaugurated the 1969 Woodstock Music Festival with what may well still be the largest-ever communal chant of the sacred syllable Om. Lilias studied briefly with the surgeon-turned-yogi Sri Brahmananda Sarasvati at his Ananda

Ashram in Monroe, New York. But it was at a nearby ashram called the Divine Life Society that Lilias found the man she calls her root teacher, Swami Chidananda. "Swamiji took a torch and lit my heart," she says. "He made me see that we are temporary boats upon this sea, that we're here to bring about our own divinity and to experience it."

Like Vishnu-devananda and Satchidananda, Chidananda had been initiated as a swami, or monk, by Swami Sivananda, the great yoga master whose Divine Life Society in Rishikesh, India, drew seekers from every corner of the world. In 1959 Sivananda sent Chidananda as an emissary to the West. When Sivananda "left his body," as yogis say, in 1963, Chidananda succeeded him as the Divine Life Society's president.

During his two-year sojourn in the West, Swami Chidananda was the frequent guest of honor at the DLS outpost in Harriman, New York, where Lilias met him. She hung on his every word.

"It was like being with Saint Francis," she says. "The dignity and inspiration of his presence just heightened the energy field of everyone around him. So here I am married, I've got two kids, and I'm flying out the door every chance I get to be with holy people. And I thought, This is difficult."

She was attending a hatha yoga class at Harriman in September 1965 when her husband called with the news that her father had died. To collect herself before driving home, Lilias went into the ashram's meditation temple and prepared to practice *tratak,* fixing the gaze to center the mind. Her eyes were drawn to a photograph on the altar of a man with the kindest eyes she had ever seen. Gazing at him, Lilias fell into a state of meditation more profound than she had imagined was possible. What struck her afterward was that she had gazed into these eyes before—as an eleven-year-old poring over the pages of *LIFE* magazine.

"In the days before television *LIFE* brought into

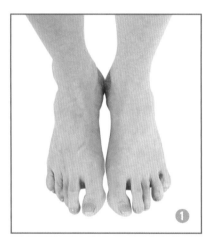
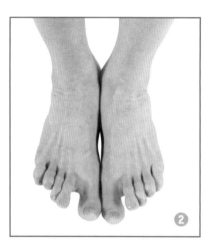
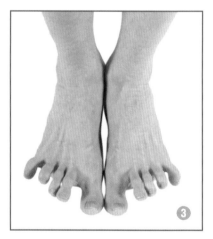

Practicing Mountain *(Tadasana)*

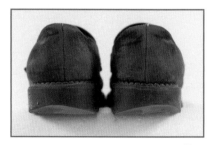

1. Notice how you stand, beginning with your feet. Roll to the outer edges of your feet ❶, then to the inner edges ❷, rock back on the heels, and forward onto the balls of your feet. Then come to stand evenly on all four corners of each foot. Lift and spread all ten toes ❸ and, starting with the pinkies, stretch each toe back out onto the floor. Extend the evenness of your feet up the calves and thighs to the alignment of the femur bones in the hip sockets. To learn how you stand on the earth, look at the soles of an old pair of your shoes ❹. Use that information to help correct rather than reinforce imbalance in your asana practice.

people's homes exactly what was going on all over the world," Lilias says. "I saw, in black and white, the horror of the Holocaust; my heart broke, seeing that at eight years old. Then, in May 1949 there was an article on this luminous teacher from India. I looked at the faces of these people looking at him, including American women in saris, and I looked at his face as he looked out at them. And that was how I met Ramana Maharshi and met him once again at Harriman—through his image, which still holds the power and electricity of this very evolved being."

Later that year Lilias was with her husband on their boat on Long Island Sound when another profound connection—or reconnection—occurred. She refers to it now as "the fiery birthing of the beloved within," but when it happened, she was awestruck and a little frightened. "Something in my chest began to just open," she says. "It felt like a thumb pressing from the inside out." So she undertook a journey to describe this indescribable feeling to the only person she knew would understand it: her teacher, Swami Chidananda, then residing at the Sivananda Yoga Center in Val Morin, Quebec.

"I wanted to leave my home, my children, everything, and do nothing but dedicate my life to God. So I took that thought and the angst it caused, and I told Swami what had happened. And he said, 'Oh, did it feel like a thumb pressing from the inside of your chest out?' Then he said, 'Lilias, you have been called by God, but you were

THE YOGA OF THE POSE: "This posture helps me to settle into my body and into my heart and into my inner teacher. It's a coming home that deepens as time goes on. With the palms pressed together and the feet together or comfortably apart, if you awaken to the *sakshin*, which means tuning into your witness self, you observe in a flash—really quickly—what you have brought to class today. Ask yourself, Where am I? Encouraging yourself to welcome rather than run from that brings you to the present moment.

"It is also beautiful to go outside and do *Tadasana*, just to feel a part of everything and that everything is a part of who you are. As a mountain, your feet are really in the earth and your head is connected to the great, expansive, never-ending blue above. It's a lovely feeling."

HOW STUDENTS COMMONLY MISS IT: "The pose is so simple that it is easy to miss and take for granted. *Tadasana* is a transition posture. It brings you from the parking lot, from the traveling to get to class on time, to this moment now. So for the type A personality who says, 'Let's get going! I want to get moving into Sun Salutations!' or 'This isn't really a posture,' it takes some maturing and understanding to realize that *Tadasana* is an important moment."

HOW TO MAKE SURE YOU CONNECT: "Like a flower that opens again and again, allow yourself to feel and be connected to your heart center. It takes a little time sometimes, because life puts up its barriers, but this is the practice. The feet, the toes—imagine them as vines that grow deep into the earth. The feet are our place of understanding. Then check into the pelvis and buckle up your seat belt (p. 29) so that you really give yourself a strong, balanced workbench from which to continue awareness up your spine. Pause at the shoulders and move them back and down.

"Once you have this wonderful long line, bring the palms of your hands together and place the base of your thumbs at your sternum. Then drop the chin slightly and bow your head so that your brain waves quiet down. Pause to give thanks to all the teachers that have gotten you to this moment in time—the difficult ones, the enlightened ones. And smile a genuine smile that slightly lifts the cheeks, affects the laugh lines around your eyes, and releases chemicals in your brain that make you feel happier and more contented. This is divine nourishment."

Mountain *(Tadasana)*

called after your marriage and not before.'" Her home and family, he told her, were the appropriate framework for her yoga *sadhana,* or practice.

Lilias left Val Morin determined to make all the pieces fit—even when her husband announced that his work made it necessary for them to relocate to Cincinnati. "Now, I knew what went on where I was living," Lilias says. "Swami was there, the ashrams were there, all my friends in my yoga classes were there"—she'd begun teaching at the Y a year and a half into her practice—"but I couldn't imagine what went on in Cincinnati, Ohio!"

As it turns out, a whole lot did. A student at the community center where Lilias began teaching was married to a television producer who thought a program on yoga might be a good idea. *Lilias, Yoga and You* started out as a local broadcast, but within eight weeks it was picked up by PBS stations

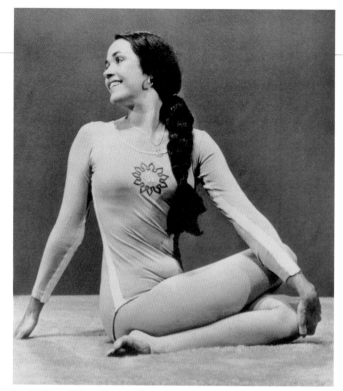

A still from Lilias Folan's first TV program, Lilias, Yoga and You, *which began airing in 1972 and was broadcast nationwide for thirteen years. Millions of Americans watched the show.*

2. To work toward correcting swayback, or lordosis ❺, draw the tailbone down toward the heels and pull the front ribs in. Practitioners with kyphosis, an excessively curved thoracic spine ❻, need to consciously draw the heads of the shoulders and the back of the head toward the wall behind them. (Step 3 may be especially useful for this type of postural imbalance.) In a well-aligned *Tadasana,* the big joints of the body form a vertical axis from the inner ankle to the jawbone ❼.

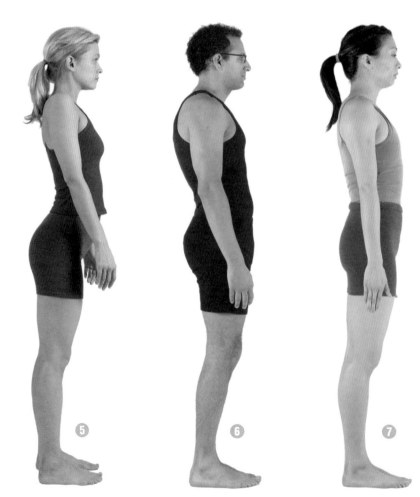

nationwide. Lilias was teaching yoga to America through the medium of television.

"The camera developed in me a style of teaching that was slow and focused," Lilias says. "Every time I sat down in front of it, I was talking to people from ten years old to eighty. And, with only a half hour, I learned that you cannot talk on and on. You have to say what you want to say, and you have got to be clear about it."

Another great lesson Lilias gave and received through television was not to become bound by an external image of the pose. "I knew from watching myself that I wasn't doing things perfectly." As a teacher, she instinctively would "tweak the asana to fit the body." But she hadn't always been as compassionate to herself. Her own desire for perfection had led to injuries she says were exacerbated by the absence of caution that typified early American asana instruction. For example, because many people practiced Shoulder Stand incorrectly, "thirty years ago you'd look around in classes and see people with a permanent bruise at the back of their neck, usually accompanied by fluid around the seventh cervical vertebra," she notes.

By the late 1970s Lilias was seeing a chiropractor weekly and was ready to give up yoga. Then she attended a workshop with Bernard Rishi, a senior teacher in the tradition of the asana master B.K.S. Iyengar (p. 50). Rishi introduced Lilias to the concept of alignment and the use of props. "He turned my practice around. I really benefited from it, and the television series benefited as well."

So Lilias's journey has been televised. Her exploration—which included a visit to India in 1973 and her honorary ordination as Swami Kavitananda by Goswami Kriyananda of Chicago's Temple of Kriya Yoga in 1998—has encompassed all aspects of the discipline, which she continues to present judiciously. "You don't have to say everything you know," she points out. "It's much more important to be an example of the change you wish to inspire. Is anything lost in the translation when we call our classes Power Yoga or Restore

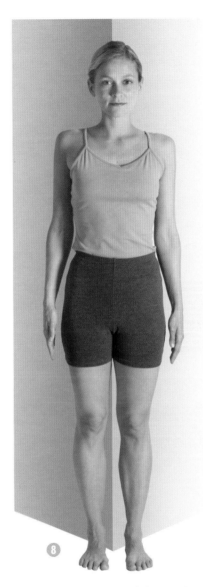

3. Lilias recommends doing *Tadasana* at a corner as a way to feel correct alignment in the pose ⑧. Stand so that the corner runs along your spine and between your buttock muscles. Rest the back of your head, your shoulders, and your heels lightly against the wall so that the shoulders roll back and the posture feels "beautiful," Lilias says. "Take your head and shoulders away, then walk away and take the wall with you."

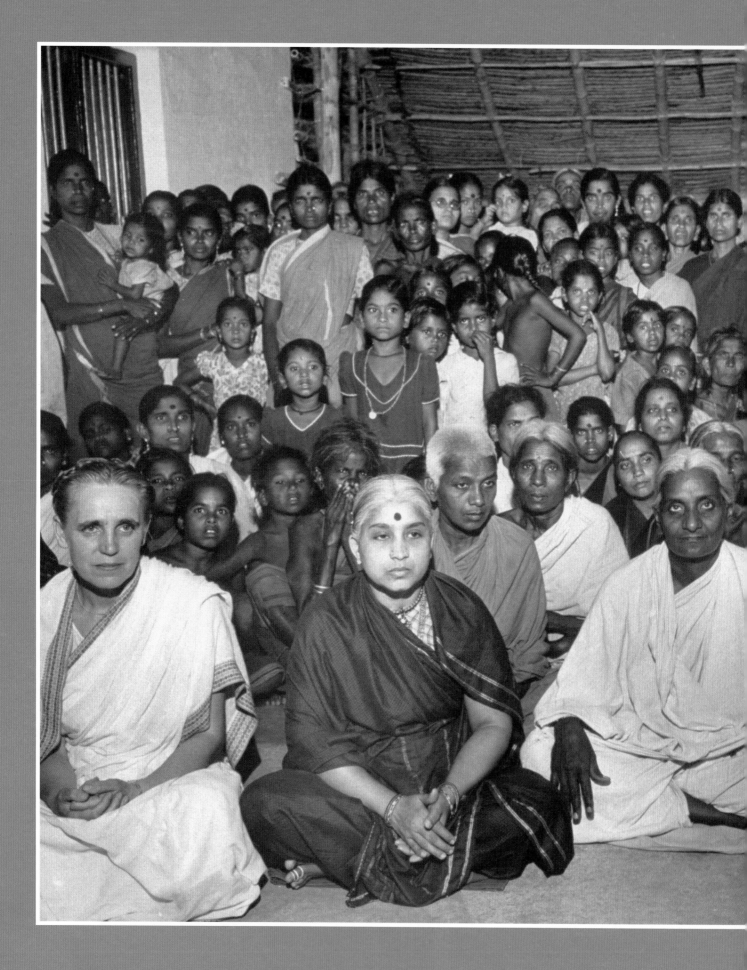

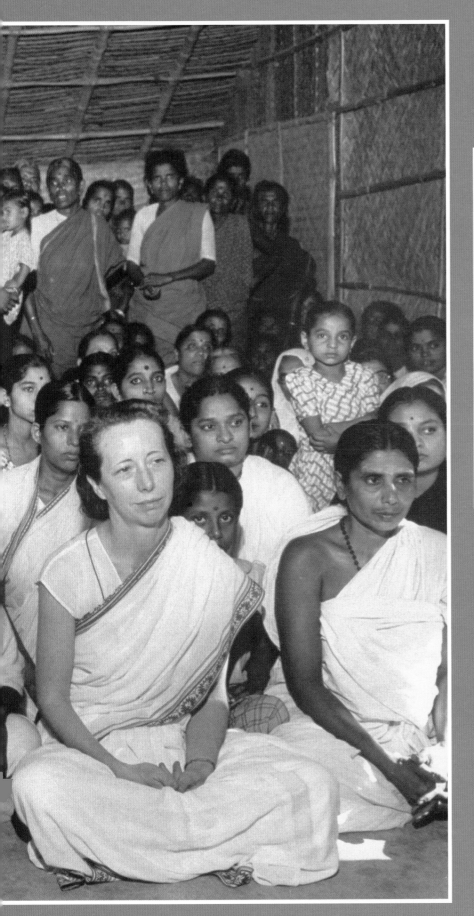

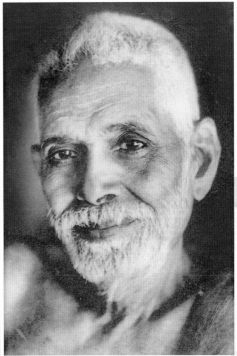

Left, the May 1949 LIFE magazine photograph of followers of the Indian sage Ramana Maharshi (above) that inspired Lilias toward the path at an early age.

and Renew? If I went to a nursing home and billed my presentation as Hatha Yoga there'd be no one there; but if I call it Rest, Relax, and Sleep everybody comes. So the answer to the question is nothing gets lost at all—as long as you know your roots."

In the mid-1970s Ram Dass was a guest on Lilias's show. He had come to yoga as an acid-dropping counterculture pioneer. She had come to it as a housewife and mother of two. But on that day, in her Cincinnati television studio, these two diverse American yogis practiced together with a single-mindedness that beamed its way into living rooms across the country. ("Look how God is using the airwaves," Ram Dass remarked.)

"So many wonderful teachers bring us to yoga—the realization that we are not just limited human beings, that we are essentially divine," Lilias says. "And what I've come to realize is that divinity, my inner friend, never left me—I had left it. The whole yoga journey has been to reconnect to that in a more mature way." For Lilias Folan, as for us all, yoga begins now, again and again.

UJJAYI: THE SOUND OF PRANA

"The citta *[consciousness] is like a chariot yoked to a team of powerful horses. One of them is breath, the other desire. The chariot moves in the direction of the more powerful animal. If breath prevails, the desires are controlled, the senses are held in check and the mind is stilled. If desire prevails, the breath is in disarray and the mind is agitated and troubled. Therefore, the yogi masters the science of the breath and by the regulation and control of the breath he controls the mind and stills its constant movement."*

—B.K.S. Iyengar, *Light on Yoga*

To attend to the breath is to practice yoga—whether you are carrying out a series of asanas or sitting still for *pranayama* or meditation. Watching the breath as it moves in and out tells us everything we need to know about the state of our mind, our heart, and our soul. If the breath is ragged or forced, we have become separated from our sense of compassion. If it is fast and shallow, we have lost our connection with the calm, deep intelligence that is our true nature.

The method of *pranayama* or breath expansion known as *ujjayi* (victory) breath lets you observe and regulate this most obvious reflection of *prana,* life-force energy. By partly closing the glottis, or back of your throat, you can hear the measured whisper of inhalations and exhalations. They should be of equal duration and variously audible—sometimes only to you, sometimes to the person next to you—but never aggressive.

Ujjayi can be employed from Sun Salutations all the way up to the last asana. (Remember to let the *pranayama* go in *Savasana,* however.) Unfortunately, the directive to "hear the breath"—a common instruction in the vigorous classes so popular in America today—has some type A practitioners growling their way through what is intended to be a contemplative practice. Ninety minutes of that leaves you far from the state of yoga.

"Ah, the widely misunderstood *ujjayi* breath," Richard Freeman says. "It's not often done well. They're struggling. They're on their way to the slaughterhouse, and they're still breathing. I try to explain that the sound of *ujjayi* breath is a mantra. You are whispering the name of your beloved. So it's a soft, pleasant thing."

Bring yourself back again and again to the quality and essence of your breath, and keep it sweet and strong, like your practice. Let it remind you who we are.

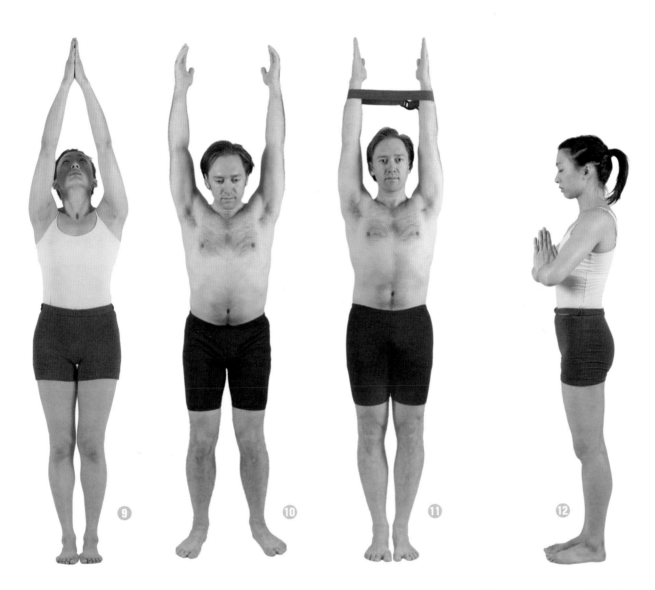

4. Feel the full measure of your mountain by reaching your arms alongside your ears, shoulder distance apart, or press the palms overhead in prayer ⑨, the second movement of the Astanga Sun Salutation A (p. 32). To make a mountain out of a molehill, typified by lazy arms and legs ⑩, hug the bones of your legs with your muscles and shoot energy through your fingertips as you draw the shoulders down toward the hips ⑪. Strap your forearms together and press out from the midline if your elbows bend due to tight or overly developed upper body musculature.

5. Once you've established your mountain, press your palms together in front of your heart ⑫. Or position the prayer as Lilias does with the top knuckle of each thumb pressed at the top of the sternum, just below the collarbones. Lilias refers to the two little indentations there as the lake of tranquillity. "With your thumbs there and the palms of your hands together, you can immediately tap into that," she says.

Sivananda-style Sun Salutation *(Surya Namaskar)*

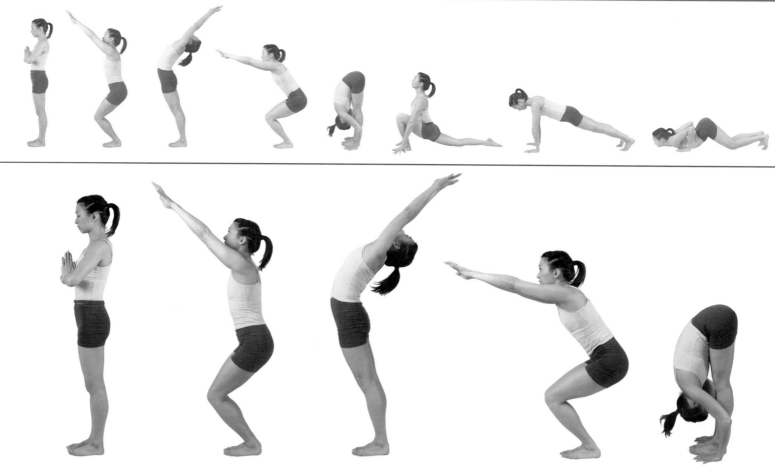

1. Stand in Mountain *(Tadasana)* with your feet together and hands in prayer in front of your heart. Exhale.

2. Inhaling, bend your knees and stretch your arms up and overhead with your thumbs hooked and fingers spread wide. Arch back from the waist with your legs straight and your neck relaxed.

3. Exhaling, fold forward into Intense Stretch *(Uttanasana)*. Press your palms into the floor, fingertips in line with toes. Bend your knees if necessary.

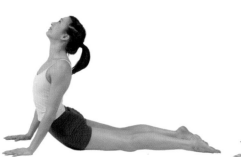

7. Inhaling, slide forward to lower your hips and arch back into Cobra *(Bhujangasana)*. Keep your legs active and shoulders down.

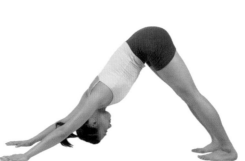

8. Exhaling, curl your toes under, raise your hips, and pivot into the inverted V of Downward-Facing Dog *(Adho Mukha Svanasana)*.

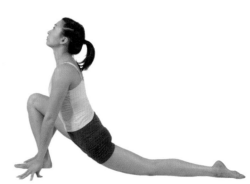

9. Inhaling, step the right foot forward between your hands. Rest the left knee on the floor and look up.

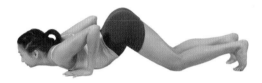

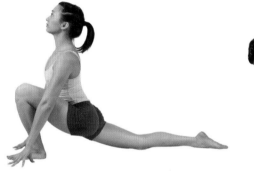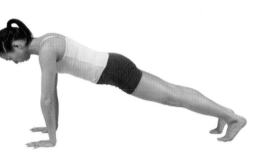

4. Inhaling, extend the right leg back and place the knee on the floor. Arch back and look up, lifting your chin.

5. Retaining the breath, bring the left leg back and support your weight on hands and toes in Plank pose.

6. Exhaling, lower your knees, chest, and chin or forehead to the floor, keeping your hips up and toes curled under.

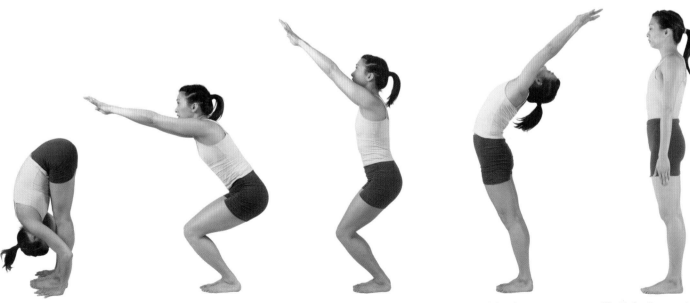

10. Exhaling, bring the left leg forward and bend over your legs with your palms pressed next to your feet.

11. Inhaling, stretch your arms forward, then up and back over your head, and bend back slowly from the waist, as in step **2**.

12. Exhaling, return to *Tadasana* with your arms alongside your body.

Richard Freeman
Intense Stretch
(Uttanasana with Trini variation)

In the modern transmission of yoga Richard Freeman is a national treasure. He casually quotes arcane scriptures as reference points when teaching the advanced practitioners who travel from far and wide to study with him. Yet he continues to instruct first-timers in his Boulder, Colorado, studio, where students slip payment, on the honor system, into an embroidered silk pouch. It's all very Eastern. It's completely Western. The breadth of Richard's experience lets him equally be both.

"At first we 'convert' to yoga and gain a new ego, as if we were trying to become little Indians—and this is understandable," Richard says. "But it's a mistake. At some point we have to look at the core teachings and find out what the real purpose of the practice is." Richard knows whereof he speaks. He has shaved his head and worn orange robes in his hometown of St. Louis, traveled in India as a *saddhu,* or seeker, presented Hindu teachings amid a brewing Islamic revolution, and sounded the depths of marriage and fatherhood. The pursuit of Self-realization, switched on early, has driven it all.

"When I was thirteen years old, I read *Walden*, by Henry David Thoreau, which is almost a mindfulness text," Richard says. "I became entranced with that whole approach to life represented by transcendentalists like Walt Whitman, who were actually the first Americans to get early translations of the Vedas and the *Bhagavad Gita* and some of the Upanishads." Richard discovered the concept of yoga as a practice separate from philosophy when he was a senior in high school. The asana book he came upon was one his mother had, called *Yoga Over Forty*. And his first teacher was a roshi at the Zen Center in Chicago. "He was the only person around with any genuine experience of yoga. The thing is, he only taught one posture: Sitting. But you know, you can't be too particular."

In 1968 Richard went off to Shimer College, then an experimental wing of the

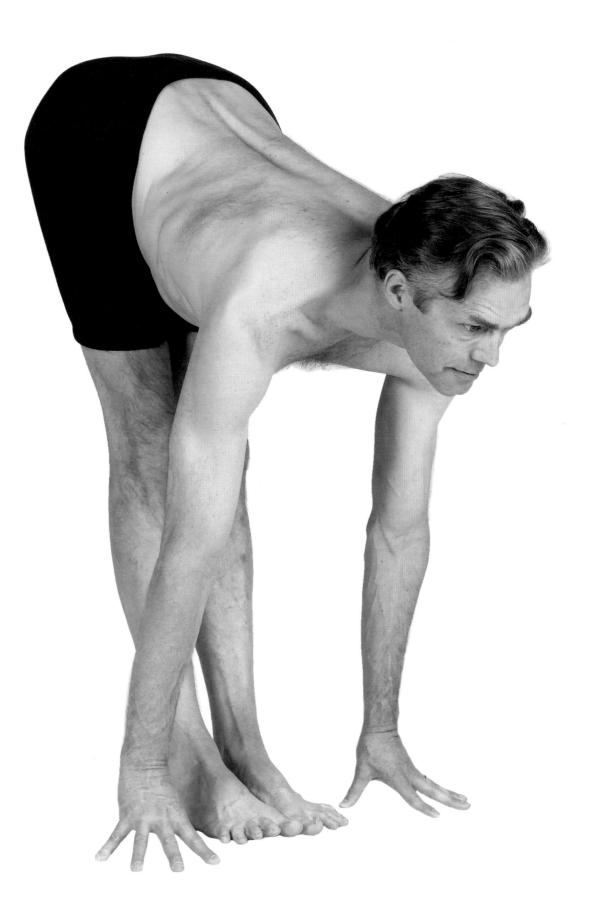

Intense Stretch *(Uttanasana* with *Trini* variation)*

THE YOGA OF THE POSE: "If you ride the wave of the breath, *Trini*—the third position in the Sun Salutation (p. 32)—is like hitting a light switch in your body. When you pull the breath up through the point above the center of your pelvic floor, it lights up alignment oppositions all along the spine and then out through the limbs."

HOW STUDENTS COMMONLY MISS IT: "It's a very energizing posture, but most people don't do it with any life. So it doesn't really have that effect. They are afraid, I think, of feeling that deep into the body, so they won't straighten the spine—or if they do, they hyperextend it. And they tend not to ground the feet well or to lift the skin or the muscles of the legs brightly."

HOW TO MAKE SURE YOU CONNECT: "Drink a cup of coffee. Or better yet, become aware of what you're feeling so that you're not so much obsessed with what you're getting out of the practice or with how you look to others, but you're really paying attention to patterns and sensation and breath in the core of the body.

"Lift your head and straighten your back. If you cannot do this with straight legs, bend your knees and take your hands off the floor. Either way, stretch out your tail feathers by lifting the buttock muscles, which increases the inward spiraling of legs and sets the pubic bone way back between the upper thighs. That invites an internal counteraction that will reveal to you your pelvic floor, which is the base of all poses."

Practicing Intense Stretch *(Uttanasana* with *Trini* variation)*

1. *Uttanasana* means "intense stretch," and while your stretch may not look as intense as that of the person next to you, the deliberateness of the work should be the same. In the Astanga-style Sun Salutations the common instruction is to "swan dive" forward over straight legs and place your palms next to your feet ❶. But as you begin your practice, this may not be possible. So bend your knees as necessary to lay your palms on the floor ❷.

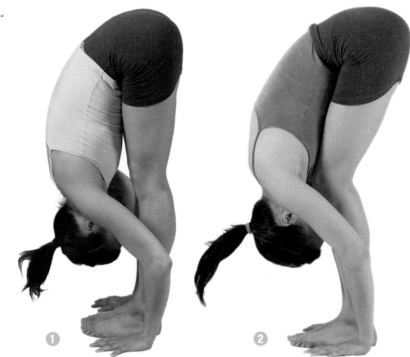

❶ ❷

University of Chicago. As part of his physical education credits Richard taught yoga classes, having discovered another asana manual, a book from India that taught *bandhas* (p. 29), *kriyas* or cleansing practices, and basic yoga poses. Then, back in St. Louis, Richard encountered a robed man chanting on the streets and joined him and the town's sole other devotee to become a Hare Krishna—"but not a normal one," he says. "When they started pushing books and magazines, I left. It didn't seem to me to be what it was about."

Richard left St. Louis to study the roots of the Krishna movement in India. He stayed a year in Brindaban, where the avatar Krishna is said to have manifested, and then traveled the subcontinent to Southeast Asia, "staying in all manner of ashrams. I studied asana by watching *saddhus* who did it," he says.

After nearly four years in India chance brought Richard to prerevolutionary Iran, where he taught yoga to the royal family and to less wealthy clients, a number of whom were Sufis. "I became quite good at relating yogic information cross-culturally, juxtaposing the Hindu or Indian teachings with Islam," he says. "You had to be very careful with what you said."

It was 1974 when Richard finally took his first yoga class—in Tehran, of all places, from an Indian woman who taught Iyengar Yoga. Richard found the style static and mechanical. But the next year, on a visit to India, he met B.K.S. Iyengar himself, who "was most radical and subtle," Richard says. He became strongly influenced by the master, studying with him in Pune and later whenever Iyengar came to the States.

In September 1978 the Islamic revolution

2. Develop stability and extension by folding in half with your feet hip distance apart. (Note that this is only six to eight inches.) Wrap your right fingers around your left elbow and your left fingers around your right elbow, and let your head dangle between your upper arms. Bend your knees to release the spine ❸, then stretch the sitting bones to the ceiling and lengthen the crown of the head toward the floor ❹.

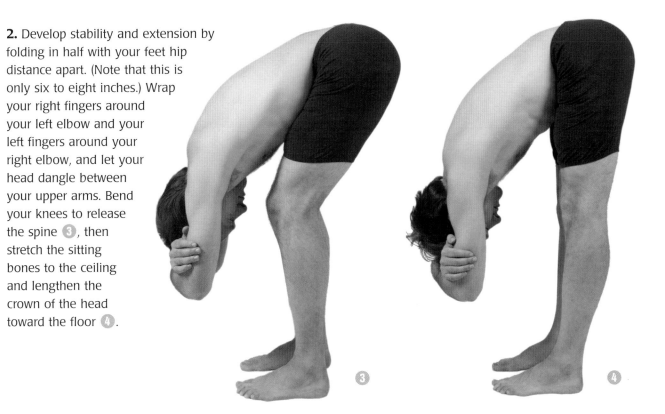

began in Iran. Richard recalls "rivers of blood in the street" in the two months before he finally fled the country in what today seems like a wildly delayed departure. "We would never do what we do if we knew what was down the line," Richard says.

Eventually Richard moved to Boulder, Colorado, where he opened his yoga studio. In 1987 he attended a workshop given in Montana by the man Richard describes as his current teacher, the Astanga Yoga guru K. Pattabhi Jois. Richard had tried out Jois's method on his own and was proficient at all the individual poses. But practicing the

entire first form of the Astanga Yoga posture flow, known as the primary series, "required a level of physical fitness that was surprising," he says. "And it was much more intense with him. It's just endlessly intense—particularly if he's standing right next to you."

During that workshop, Jois took Richard and one or two others to the highly challenging second and third series of Astanga Yoga methodology. But something far beyond asana was being transmitted. "Because I had an interest in Sanskrit and the internal practices of yoga, he shared much of that with me in the first week I knew him and when I

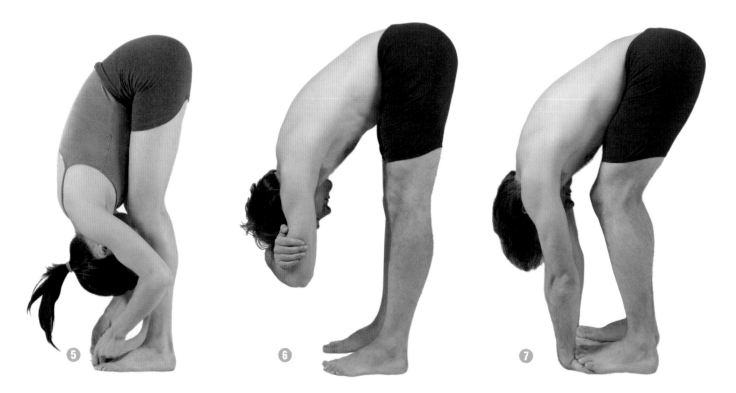

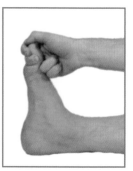

3. Two poses included in the Astanga Yoga series deepen our comprehension of standing forward bends. For Big Toe pose *(Padangusthasana)* ⑤, grasp the big toes with the first and second finger of each hand in "yogic toe lock" (inset). If you cannot do this with straight legs, bend your knees, or simply take hold of opposite elbows ⑥. Hand to Foot pose *(Pada Hastasana)* ⑦ provides an excellent lesson regardless of your degree of hamstring flexibility. Slip your palms under your feet till the toes reach the wrist creases, then straighten your legs as best you can. Wherever you are in the pose is exactly where you should be, so experience *santosha*, contentment, here and work the posture with kind intensity by lifting the sitting bones to the ceiling and releasing the head and neck.

was in India with him later on," Richard says. "I was primed for it."

Richard's perspective on the guru-disciple relationship is singularly honed. "I went through a bunch of them, so I don't consider gurus the way many people do. It takes away one's intelligence and cuts off a genuine relationship to put them on pedestals. That's the old 'transference' of psychoanalysis. I don't have issues with my father anymore, so I don't need a father substitute."

Does Richard play that role unwittingly to the myriad American *saddhus* who flock to study with

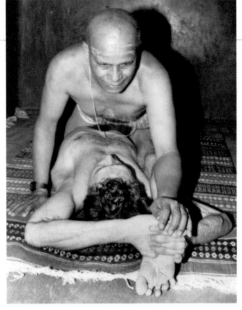

Richard being adjusted by K. Pattabhi Jois in Mysore, India, in 1987.

him each year? "Oh, yeah," he says. "But I try always to give it back to the student from day one, to not make them dependent on me. The actual guru is inside, in your own heart."

Although the primary series Richard recommends most is the ancient texts of the Upanishads—"They point out the possibility of actually gaining the insight that can give us freedom"—he insists that our truest understandings will be homegrown. "The great opportunity as yoga is transplanted from India to the West is to separate it from the cultural baggage and bring it

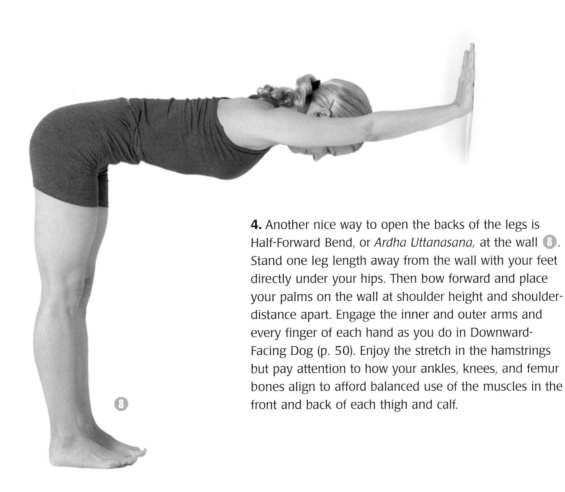

4. Another nice way to open the backs of the legs is Half-Forward Bend, or *Ardha Uttanasana,* at the wall ❽. Stand one leg length away from the wall with your feet directly under your hips. Then bow forward and place your palms on the wall at shoulder height and shoulder-distance apart. Engage the inner and outer arms and every finger of each hand as you do in Downward-Facing Dog (p. 50). Enjoy the stretch in the hamstrings but pay attention to how your ankles, knees, and femur bones align to afford balanced use of the muscles in the front and back of each thigh and calf.

Intense Stretch *(Uttanasana* with *Trini* variation)*

into our own experience," Richard says. "It's not 'getting religion.' Today, there are ultra-right-wing fundamentalist groups affecting Hinduism, and there's no reason for us coming from this culture to get caught in that. To actually look at what we're doing when we adopt the practice, to go into how the mind works through meditation—that's what's going to make our yoga successful."

Has the highly popular Astanga Yoga method, with its sweat-inducing pace of poses taught in the same order in gyms and studios nationwide, increasingly come to define American yoga? "Well, it's franchisable," Richard notes. "But at a certain point ideals meet reality. You won't find two teachers who are the same. They can dress like the guru, try to talk like him, and still it's impossible to replicate the form exactly. And right in that difficulty, where the map is not the territory, the potential for yoga is there."

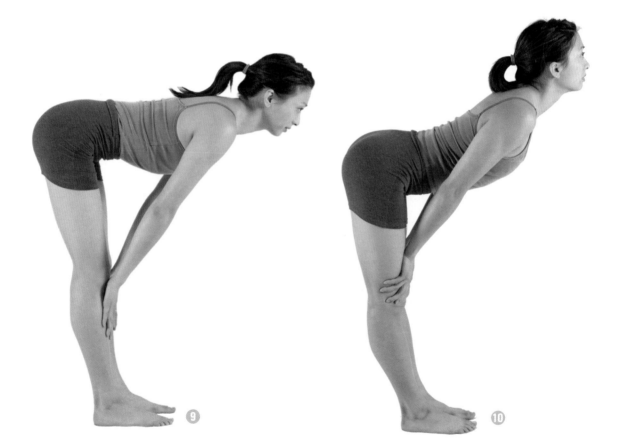

5. Take this same basic shape and intelligence into *Trini,* the *Uttanasana* variation Richard Freeman is demonstrating. If you cannot keep the fingertips next to your feet with straight legs, raise your hands off the floor or up to the shins ⑨. Avoid hyperextending the backs of the knees and the spine, as Richard warns against ⑩. Keep the spine long by expanding through the front of the body. And to place the femur correctly in the hip socket, "microbend" the knee, Richard recommends, which also tones the hamstrings so they don't "turn off," he says. "It makes an incredible difference to your joints in the long run. You can just pull yourself to pieces with yoga!"

LOCKING TO FLOW: ASTANGA, ASTANGA YOGA, AND BANDHAS

The term *astanga,* which means eight limbs in Sanskrit, is often a source of confusion for neophytes. The nomenclature comes from the *Yoga Sutras* (p. 56), a Sanskrit text dating to around 200 C.E. that codified the already millennia-old teachings of yoga philosophy. But the word is also the name of a style of practice popularized by K. Pattabhi Jois that he learned as a young man from his teacher, T. Krishnamacharya.

Jois, a Brahmin, or upperclass Hindu, was reluctant to teach the first American who sought him out in the late 1960s. Now his tours of America draw ever increasing numbers of acolytes who want to study with the guru of Astanga Yoga. The practice is a muscular ballet of poses linked by gymnastic jumpings and carried out at a nearly aerobic pace. Each fixed series—from the first, or "primary series," to the prohibitively challenging, rarely done sixth—covers the bases with regard to asanas and is meant to be meted out by a certified instructor according to each student's level of development. Done well, it is a marvel to experience and to behold. Done inappropriately, it can be downright dangerous. Jois calls the practice *yoga cikitsa* or yoga therapy. But Astanga Yoga as widely practiced today is far different from the *cikitsa* prescribed by Krishnamacharya's son, the Viniyoga master T.K.V. Desikachar, or by Desikachar's longtime student Gary Kraftsow, who continues the tradition here in America (p. 152).

Astanga Yoga's intense athleticism seems to suit our national temperament, however, and there is much to be said for doing the same practice on a regular basis. Over time practitioners can dispassionately watch their mental and physical advancement through the increasingly complex series. The style has forever changed American yoga, much of which now bears Astanga's imprint to varying degrees.

In addition to *ujjayi* breathing (p. 18), Astanga Yoga is founded on the subtle, often grossly perceived *bandhas,* or locks, of yoga. *Mula bandha* (root lock) is frequently described as the lifting of the pelvic floor or perineum, the muscular tissue between the anus and genitals. *Uddiyana bandha* (flying-up lock) is the contraction from the anus to the diaphragm. And *jalandhara bandha* (chin lock) is when the spine is held tall and the chin is lowered to the crook of the neck.

All traditions use the *bandhas* selectively— most often for breath expansion practices—but Astanga Yoga practitioners maintain *mula bandha* throughout the practice. "When done correctly *mula bandha* really starts producing yogic states of mind," Richard says. "You're attending to it, like a deity, so it's different from 'doing it' or 'squeezing it.' A clenched butt is not it."

Lilias Folan learned long ago to couch such bald anatomical instruction in terms palatable to her television viewers. To "buckle up your seat belt," as she phrases it, "point the tailbone down toward the heels and pull the muscles behind your abdomen and some of the perineum upward."

And John Friend (p. 94) teaches *bandhas* in a way that reflects his ecumenical background and style. "*Bandha* is not like a lock in a door," he says. "It's more a lock in a navigation system like the Erie Canal. When you're in India, out in the country, the farmers take pieces of wood and stick them in the ground to help navigate the waters to crops in different parts of the field. Those are called *bandhas.* So you can create energy locks through the whole of the body—from the pelvic floor to the floor of the mouth. Like psychic diaphragms, they allow a channeling of the energy. And like cheesecloth, they catch the gross impurities as the divine energy moves through."

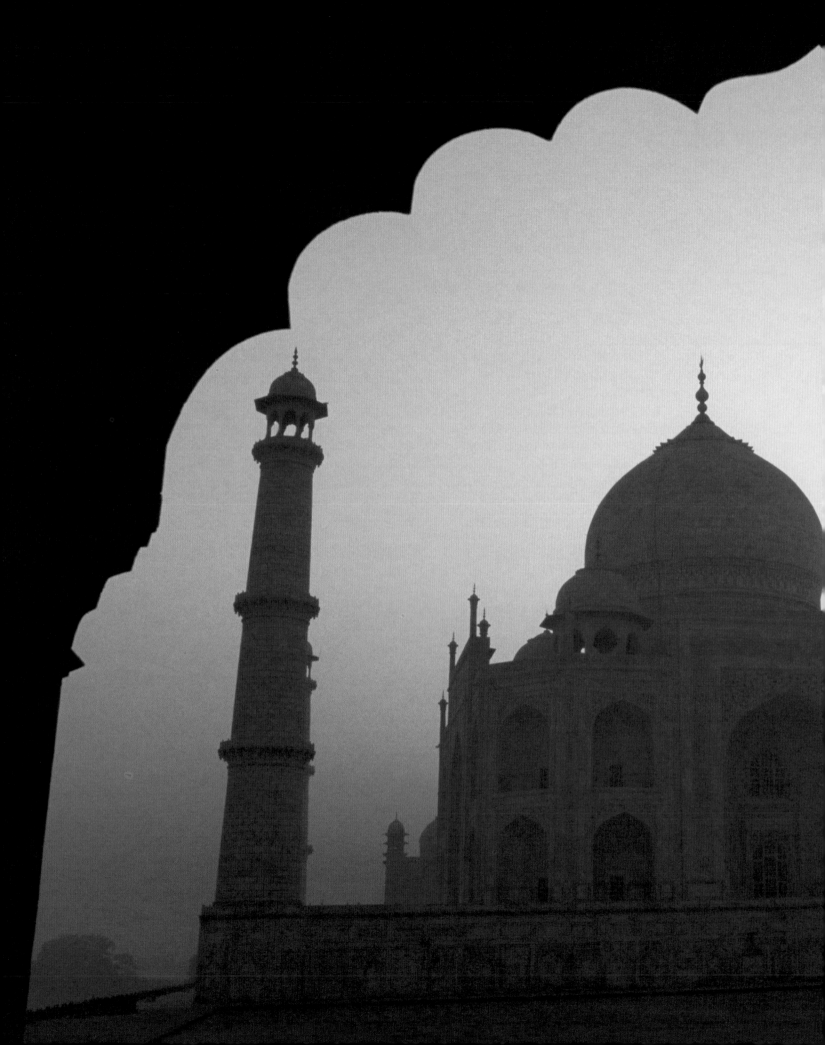

PASSAGE TO INDIA

Lo, soul, seest thou not God's purpose from the first?
The earth to be spann'd, connected by network,
The races, neighbors, to marry and be given in marriage,
The oceans to be cross'd, the distant brought near,
The lands to be welded together.

A worship new I sing,
You captains, voyagers, explorers, yours,
You engineers, you architects, machinists, yours,
You, not for trade or transportation only,
But in God's name, and for thy sake O soul.

Passage to more than India!
Are thy wings plumed indeed for such far flights?
O soul, voyagest thou indeed on voyages like those?
Disportest thou on waters such as those?
Soundest below the Sanscrit and the Vedas?
Then have thy bent unleash'd.

Passage, immediate passage! the blood burns in my veins!
Away O soul! hoist instantly the anchor!

Cut the hawsers—haul out—shake out every sail!
Have we not stood here like trees in the ground long enough?
Have we not grovel'd here long enough, eating and drinking like mere brutes?
Have we not darken'd and dazed ourselves with books long enough?

Sail forth—steer for the deep waters only,
Reckless O soul, exploring, I with thee, and thou with me,
For we are bound where mariner has not yet dared to go,
And we will risk the ship, ourselves and all.

O my brave soul!
O farther farther sail!
O daring joy, but safe! are they not all the seas of God?
O farther, farther, farther sail!

—Excerpted from *Leaves of Grass*, Walt Whitman

Astanga-style Sun Salutation A *(Surya Namaskar A)*

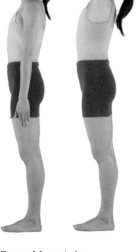

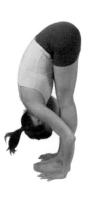

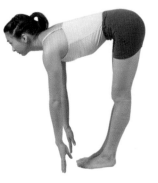

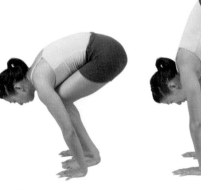

1. From Mountain *(Tadasana),* inhale as you circle your arms out and up overhead in a prayer.

2. Exhale and dive forward into Intense Stretch *(Uttanasana)* with palms alongside feet.

3. Rise to your fingertips, lengthen the spine and look up in Third Step *(Trini).*

4. Exhale and jump back into Four-Limbed Staff *(Chaturanga Dandasana).*

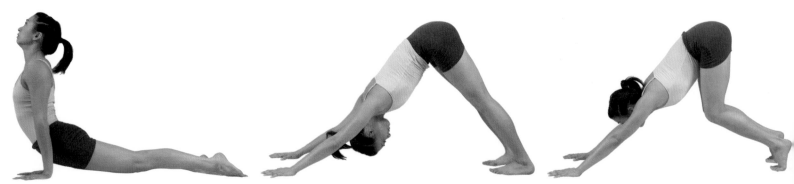

5. Inhale to Upward-Facing Dog *(Urdhva Mukha Svanasana).*

6. Exhale to Downward-Facing Dog *(Adho Mukha Svanasana).* Stay five breaths.

7. Bend the knees, lift the heels, gaze forward, and exhale.

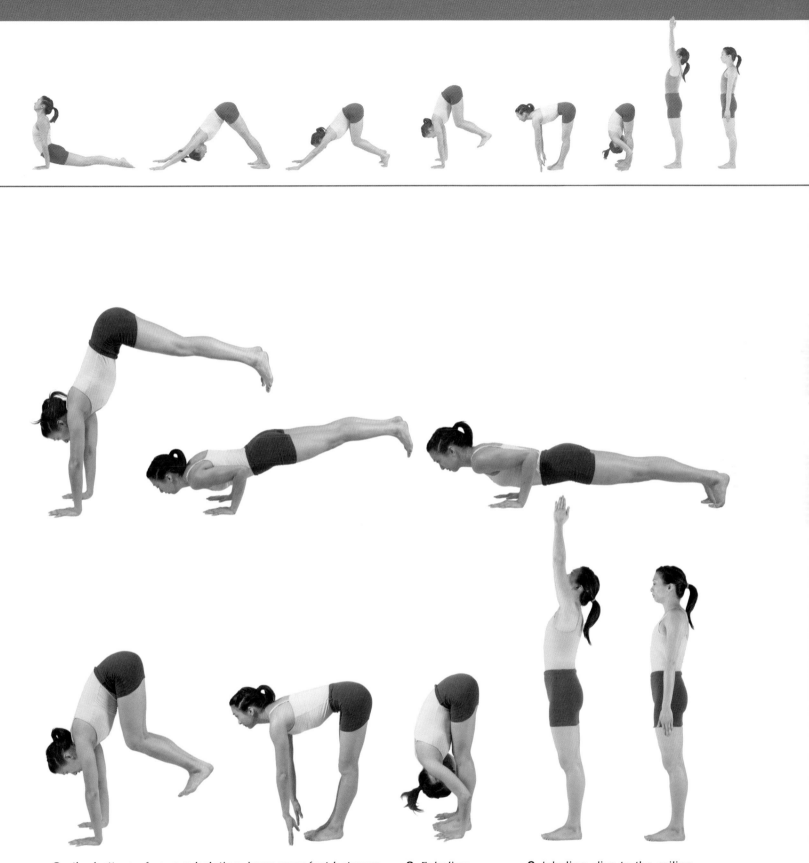

On the bottom of your exhalation, jump your feet between your hands. (Some teachers instruct you to jump forward as you inhale. See what works best for you.) Then inhale, rise to your fingertips, and look up.

8. Exhaling, bow forward into Intense Stretch (Uttanasana).

9. Inhaling, dive to the ceiling and press your palms overhead, then exhale and come to stand in Tadasana.

Beryl Bender Birch
Four-Limbed Staff
(Chaturanga Dandasana)

Like most Americans, Beryl Bender Birch was raised on the concept that the body and mind are disconnected realms. Her Presbyterian-Methodist upbringing had impressed on her that "humans were down here, and God was up there," she says. Her mother's death when Beryl was fifteen caused her to contemplate these weighty issues early and hard. Theology was the stuff of dinnertime conversation with her father, a Ph.D. chemist and former debating team captain with strong religious convictions he expressed with scientific logic. So Beryl entered college as a physics major and along the way switched to philosophy, which to her made perfect sense. "I had an unshakable notion that these things were supposed to be together," she says.

Her introduction to yoga was through *The World's Religions,* by Huston Smith, a text in the comparative religion class she took at Syracuse University in 1962. In his section on

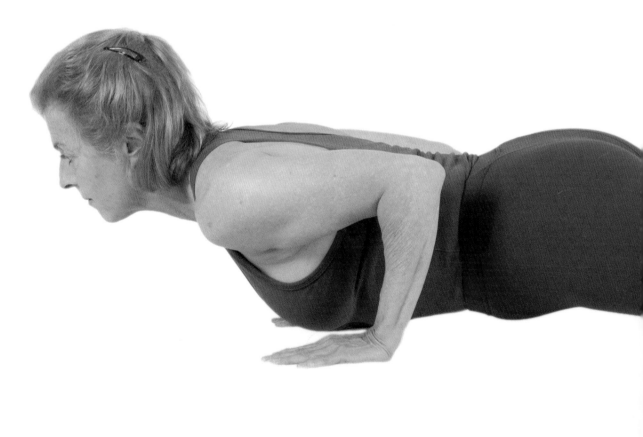

THE YOGA OF THE POSE: "You're like a laser beam of *prana* from the tip of your head to the tip of your toes. You're supercharged. It's a focused, steadying posture that builds strength, self-esteem, breath, heat, purification, and, ultimately, transformation. It teaches you where you're too spread out in your life and where you're stuck, where you're too rigid and need more fluidity, and where you're too sloppy and need to pull it in a little.

"It's interesting: When you're not good at it, it's difficult, it's unpleasant. But as you get more familiar with it, it becomes just a portion of practice; it's not good or bad but just a step on a path, a place you pass through that develops strength and heat and power. So the practice is an analogy for life. There are portions you cruise through and portions that are really difficult. The minute you get comfortable someplace, things are going to change. When you're uncomfortable someplace, hang in there, because that will change, too. In that way *Chaturanga* teaches you dispassion, or *vairagya*."

HOW STUDENTS COMMONLY MISS IT: "Because they're not strong enough. They have too much *sukha* [easefulness] and not enough *sthira* [steadiness]. They have to tighten up their act a little bit, trim it down, tone it up—but gradually. If you are sloppy in *Chaturanga*, so your shoulders hyperextend up around your ears and you sink into your low back, you'll injure yourself.

"Other people might be too strong, too rigid. They can do *Chaturanga* because they've done weight lifting or they're athletic. But they're too *sthira*, not enough *sukha*; so when it comes to Up and Down Dog, their shoulders are so bound up they can't move the spine freely."

HOW TO MAKE SURE YOU CONNECT: "Practice. Practice is the teacher. Weight-bearing exercise strengthens bones and muscles and helps create circulation in joints, so it's an especially good posture for women to learn to do—but not unto itself, only as part of a sequence.

"Athletes come to me all the time and say, 'What move can I do to fix this or strengthen that?' and I say none. You have to do the whole practice; it's a synergistic, therapeutic system. If you're in a hurry, yoga is not the right path for you. *Chaturanga*, like all the postures, needs to be taught slowly and carefully. You have to use your knees in the beginning and develop your strength in the posture until it is sleek and sharp, until you look like a four-limbed stick.

"*Chaturanga* is very therapeutic for developing neutral posture of the spine and for strengthening the shoulders, but only if you do it with correct alignment. To quote my friend David Williams"—another American yoga master in the Astanga Yoga tradition—"'If it hurts, you're doing it wrong.'"

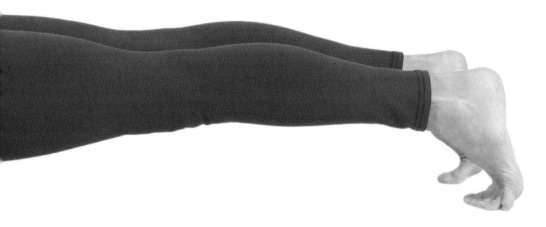

Hinduism, Smith describes the eight-limbed path of Astanga Yoga (p. 56) as "psychophysical exercise," which interested Beryl keenly. By 1971 she was living in Los Angeles—then the "hotbed of the human potential movement," as she calls it—and working at the Biofeedback Research Institute, where "lo and behold," she says, "I was witnessing the marriage of technology and consciousness."

Beryl joined the hordes of people in southern California who were exploring their consciousness in every conceivable way. "We were sitting in multiple wave oscillators, drinking gold water, which we made from putting gold bracelets in water and setting them in the sun, and doing peyote out in the desert," she recalls. "But in my work as a researcher, by using EEG biofeedback training, I began to understand that meditation is an actual measurable physiological state. It's not just some esoteric thing we think may happen. When you're approaching the proper brain wave frequencies or, as Patanjali says, when you focus on one thing, the changes are documentable."

In the fall of 1972 two pieces of news from the East Coast affected Beryl's pursuits. Her father wrote to say that he was dying of cancer, and a friend in New York phoned to announce that a great guru had come from India whom she needed to meet right away. Beryl journeyed to New Jersey to spend Christmas with her father. She hoped to sway him toward the alternative medicine practices she was convinced might heal him, but she was unsuccessful. During the visit, she traveled to New York City to attend a lecture by the founder of the Jain Meditation International Center, Munishree Chitrabhanu.

"By this point I'd already met Dr. Mishra, who became Sri Brahmananda Sarasvati. I'd met Swami Vishnu-devananda. I'd been studying high Tibetan meditation with Chögyam Trungpa Rinpoche. But with this man I definitely had a *shaktipat* experience—a white light beam connecting me to him. When he finished speaking, I felt as though somebody had come along with a buzz saw and cut out a circle of bone right over my heart *chakra,* and it just opened like a trapdoor. I had this amazing understanding about death and my father and what was happening, and all of a sudden tears were pouring out of my eyes."

A year earlier, Beryl had literally stumbled upon her first hatha yoga experience in 1971 en route to a lecture being given by Ram Dass at U.C.L.A. "I was running up some steps, and I tripped and sat down. There right in front of me was a flyer for a yoga class," she says. It was a Kundalini class, taught by Yogi Bhajan (p. 70), which she attended the very next night. "We did a lot of cat and cow exercises and wild heavy breathing," she says. "I don't remember having any out-of-body experiences there, but I remember the Indian food. Right next door was where Yogi Bhajan lived with his many devotees, and when we

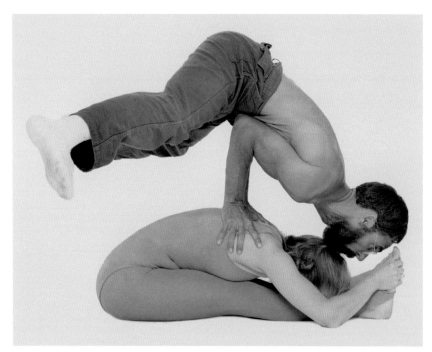

Beryl with her first Astanga Yoga teacher, Norman Allen, in 1981.

Practicing Four-Limbed Staff *(Chaturanga Dandasana)*

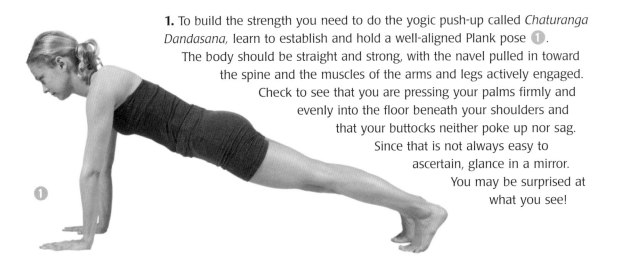

1. To build the strength you need to do the yogic push-up called *Chaturanga Dandasana,* learn to establish and hold a well-aligned Plank pose ❶. The body should be straight and strong, with the navel pulled in toward the spine and the muscles of the arms and legs actively engaged. Check to see that you are pressing your palms firmly and evenly into the floor beneath your shoulders and that your buttocks neither poke up nor sag. Since that is not always easy to ascertain, glance in a mirror. You may be surprised at what you see!

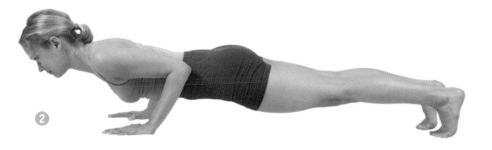

2. From Plank, bend your elbows straight back and slowly lower down until your upper arms are parallel to the floor ❷. "If you can't hold it, put your knees down ❸ and do the negative part of the push-up by slowly lowering down from there, eventually dropping your chest between your thumbs," Beryl advises. "If you do this every day, it won't take long—maybe a month—to build to *Chaturanga.*"

Four-Limbed Staff *(Chaturanga Dandasana)*

3. When practitioners lack the strength to bend their elbows straight back, as Beryl demonstrates, they collapse into the pose in a variety of ways. "Some students hyperextend their shoulders and sag into it, running *Chaturanga* and Up Dog together," she notes ❹. Others drop down too low until their chest drops below their elbows ❺. If you repeatedly do *Chaturanga* with your shoulder joints a half inch off the floor, your upper arms at a 45-degree angle to the floor, your butt up in the air, and your elbows poking up like a grasshopper's ❻ you will damage your acromioclavicular or AC joint."

4. To show the final alignment of the pose to students who cannot yet attain it, David Life sometimes teaches *Chaturanga* at the wall ❼. Stand with your toes up the wall and the balls of your feet on the floor, feet no wider than hip-width apart. Place your hands on the wall so that your wrists and elbows are in line. Lift your chin so that it is parallel to the floor, then press down into your heels and bring your body parallel to the wall. "Pull your shoulder blades down your back, squeeze the buttock muscles, and draw in the navel and front ribs at the same time," David says. "Nothing should touch the wall except the toes and hands."

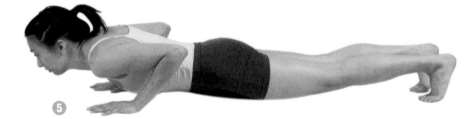

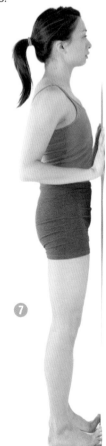

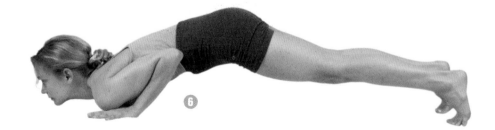

started class, they would start cooking dinner. They would be sautéing cumin and coriander and cardamom and chilis and mustard seeds, and we would go wild with the smell."

She connected a bit more deeply with the Sivananda style of practice and wound up living at the L.A. ashram for six months in 1972. But none of the asana or meditation practices she had encountered moved her as intensely as Jainism, an ancient Indic religion that uses meditation, mantra, and scripture to promote the yogic precept of *ahimsa,* nonharming or reverence for life. Chitrabhanu was the first Jain master to come to the West. "If you take the vows of Jain monks, you have to walk everywhere, because conveyances are *himsic* [harming]," Beryl says. "He got thrown out of the church for coming, but he did anyway, because he felt he had been instructed to bring these teachings to the West."

Throughout the next decade Beryl continued to study with Chitrabhanu, even importing him to California, where she "toured" him, along with his wife and baby, around to the various schools of yoga she had begun to explore. Beryl, in turn, journeyed to India in 1974. She lived with Jain families, spent a month in silence with Jain nuns, and photographed and wrote about the Kumba Mehla—the nationwide pilgrimage to the Ganges made by seekers in India every twelve years—for the magazine *East-West Journal.* When she returned to the States, she moved to the Rocky Mountain ski town of Winter Park, Colorado, where she began teaching Sivananda-style yoga flavored with visualization and behavior modification techniques. And she kept traveling east to practice with Chitrabhanu.

Beryl says, "Chitrabhanu was definitely my guru for a lot of years, but I didn't go quite as deep into that route as some. Everybody was changing their names and wearing white clothes and throwing away their jewelry and staying in marriages they didn't really want to stay in or practicing celibacy they didn't really want to practice. People

would ask, 'What's your name?' And I would say, 'Beryl.' And they'd say, 'What's your spiritual name?' And I'd say, 'Beryl.'"

That straightforward approach to things spiritual made Beryl's teaching as popular with skiers in Colorado as it did with runners in New York, where in 1981 she was named wellness director of the New York City Road Runners Club. It also kept her on an even keel that same year when Chitrabhanu's center, where she'd been asked to head up a yoga teacher training program, imploded in sexual scandal.

Like so many Indian yoga masters faced with the temptations of the American dream, "Chitrabhanu succumbed," Beryl says. "But for everybody who encounters a teacher, whatever that teacher ends up being or doing or saying is exactly what that person needed to learn. Some people deify the guru, so when they catch the guru eating chocolate chip cookies in the closet, they go back to wearing lipstick, smoking pot, and drinking wine. But who did you give up all that stuff for in the first place? For yourself and for your personal *tapas* [austerity], or for somebody else you're devastated to find is just like you?"

Being on hand to teach at the Jain center at that time proved to be Beryl's segue to the next and most important practice she would encounter: the Astanga style of hatha yoga. That February she attended a demonstration by Norman Allen, the first Western student of K. Pattabhi Jois. The radical fluidity of his movement through a linked, nonstop series of classic asanas was like nothing Beryl had seen, and she loved it. Here was the very incarnation of "The Hard & the Soft," the name she'd chosen for her yoga program seven years earlier, culled from a Zen proverb that states, "Only when you can be extremely soft and pliable can you be extremely hard and strong." For the next two years Beryl studied with Allen at six a.m. every day the moon wasn't new or full. (Astanga Yoga reserves those days for rest and contemplation.)

The system transformed her practice, her

teaching, and her life. By 1987 she and her husband, Thom, had begun studying with Jois himself, joining the still small number of Astangis who flocked to study with the master on his tour of the western United States. "Then, like now, he spoke very little English," Beryl says. "He could say, 'You take it more coffee.' He'd come sit on your back and say, 'Oh, you breathing, not fearing.' He loved Bruce Lee movies, so we'd sit and watch them every night. We used to chauffeur him and his wife around in my '82 Honda station wagon with two of our dogs." It was as fun as it was intense, she says, and Jois's tutelage took her to a whole new level.

Back in New York, Beryl continued to teach the method, which in 1989 she started calling Power Yoga. She originally used the name to promote classes at the New York Road Runners Club. But when she published a book in 1995 using *Power Yoga* as its title, the nomenclature drew as much initial fire as eventual imitators in the yoga world. Beryl regrets nothing.

"I thought it was a great idea then, and I still think it's a great idea," she says. "What is the objective? How do you teach this system to people at various stages of development and get them turned on? I decided if I called it Astanga Yoga, nobody would pay attention, so I called it Power Yoga. It was a way to let Westerners know this practice was a workout for body and mind. But Pattabhi Jois didn't like it. He couldn't get past the word 'power' in the title. The classical connotation of the word refers to the *siddhis,* or yogic powers, which the Sutras teach us not to pursue. To a Brahmin, such use of that word would be sacrilegious. To the male Western mind, power can mean bodybuilding, money, control. But what I was referring to was the power to conquer one's ego, the inner enemy. There is power in yoga; it isn't just soft chanting and singing and burning incense and all the preconceptions Americans had at the time.

"So I got thrown out of the church. It was painful, but it was good—because until you are forced from the group, you don't learn to stand on your own two feet." Beryl remains faithful to the Astanga Yoga system; and she finds the teachings she received from Jois have only deepened with age. "He would always say, 'Take it practice, all is coming,' which I now realize may be the most brilliant thing anybody's ever said. It's like when you read Patanjali's sole direct reference to asana (p. 178) —*sthira-sukham-asanam,* 'The Hard & the Soft'—and suddenly you realize that's all there is."

Beryl's early studies with the Tibetan meditation master Chögyam Trungpa Rinpoche imparted another lesson that has flowered with time. "He taught strict, precise meditation techniques. He would tell us it was very important that we do it in this particular sequence and in this particular way. Just when we got it down, new students would come in, and he would teach them something totally different. He told them that it was just as important that they did it that particular way. Then we would argue about who was right. It took me a long time to realize he did this intentionally. He wanted his students arguing about what was right so we would learn it's not about right or wrong, but about appropriateness. I see young practitioners today arguing about asana form. 'Should my hands be this way or this way? Does the left leg come in first or the right leg? Which one is *right?*'

"I was that way. We all want to know, 'When do you get really good?' Really good is three hours in one posture. The rest of it is just practice. So whether you do it at a gym, in a health club, or at the holiest place on earth, don't have an attitude about it. Get to work. That's plain English, but it's classic yoga." Beryl Bender Birch's teachings are resolutely both.

5. Beyond strengthening the arms, back, and shoulders, *Chaturanga,* like many asanas, tones the abdominal organs. As is the case in many asanas, that benefit is aided by strong abdominal muscles. Boat pose *(Navasana)* 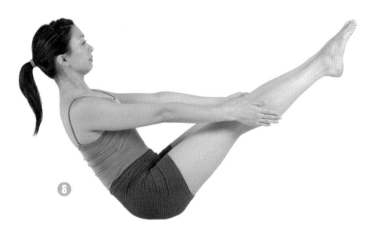, part of the Astanga primary series, is one of hatha yoga's best abdominal strengtheners. To move into the pose, lift your arms and legs into a V and gaze at your toes as you balance on your sitting bones with your torso extended parallel to the floor and to each other. If your shoulders and lower back collapse in the pose, bend your knees until your shins are parallel to the floor and lift your heart from there, breathing calmly and strongly.

6. Try moving dynamically from *Navasana* to *Ardha Navasana* (Half Boat) 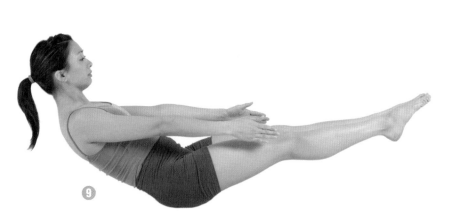, lowering as you exhale and lifting back up as you inhale. Or hold the pose and, as is often done in the Kundalini tradition, use *Ardha Navasana* to practice the rapid sniffing inhalations and exhalations of Breath of Fire (p. 74). "The concentrated energy the posture creates in the thigh muscles, the base of the spine, and the abdominal region is further stimulated when we add Breath of Fire," Krishna Kaur says. "Because we're moving the breath through with such rapid motion, pushing more oxygen in and toxins out, we can sustain the posture longer, providing a greater opportunity to get more of its strengthening benefits." One and a half to two minutes is optimal, she says.

Erich Schiffmann

Cobra
(Bhujangasana)

In his early teens Erich Schiffmann set out to discover yoga. His journey has been singularly auspicious. "I lucked out somehow, and all I was doing was following my nose," Erich says. "One thing led to the next almost magically."

That magic was not yet apparent on his twelfth birthday, when Erich's older brother, Karl, presented him with a yoga book. He thought, What a stupid gift, put it into a drawer, and forgot about it. But three years later he rediscovered it and started "fiddling around" with poses. Soon Erich was buying yoga books for himself.

"In a health food store I saw a little blue book called *Metaphysical Meditation*, with a picture of Paramahansa Yogananda on the front," he says. "I liked the picture, and I was sort of embarrassed about buying it but went ahead and bought it anyway." The practices prescribed in its pages proved a powerful draw for the

THE YOGA OF THE POSE: "Everyone can do it. It's easy, and you can get in there deep. You can do it gently, or if someone's bendy, they can really curve. The Cobra is malleable, wiggly, writhing, snakelike, strong, slow, quick, alert—all with intensive feeling about it. It's this curving arch of energy that's intense but smooth."

HOW STUDENTS COMMONLY MISS IT: "They're a little too heady about it, not feeling-oriented enough. You can have too many ideas in advance about what you're supposed to do. That's why I like to close my eyes in Cobra. Once you close your eyes, you get into the feeling of it, and the feeling starts telling you what to do. You know where it feels right and where something needs to be changed slightly, and you just keep tweaking it from inside."

HOW TO MAKE SURE YOU CONNECT: "Go slower. Get into the breathing. And do the same thing but from different ways. Do the Cobra by coming up off the floor, sometimes get into it from Cat pose and sometimes from Dog pose, by rotating your hips backward and lowering the hips down. You end up in the same place, but coming at it from different sides makes the pose dimensional. Just doing something different feels courageous, and it gives people permission to do as the inner feeling says. One of the options will feel the best, and the skill is to do the one that feels the most right.

"Start facedown and curve up without using your arms, so you're using your back strength to lift you up. Then use your arms a little bit; then use your arms more. To go into Upward-Facing Dog, continue to move like a snake, with the whole body involved. Where people hurt themselves often in Cobra or Up Dog is by overpowering their spine with their arm strength. So use your arms, but keep the legs and spine really awake."

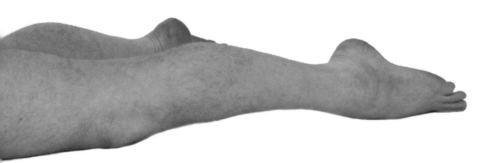

southern California boy who began to attend meditation and chanting sessions at the Self-Realization Fellowship center Yogananda established in Los Angeles back in 1924.

Paramahansa Yogananda first came to America in 1920 to address an international congress of religious leaders in Boston. His discourse on yoga, like that of Swami Vivekananda at the World's Parliament of Religions in Chicago in 1893, had tremendous impact on the men and women who heard it. Interest grew in the ancient discipline, and Yogananda stayed to teach it in America, fulfilling his guru's mandate to become a progenitor of yoga in the West. After his death in

1952 his teachings remained a beacon to many Western seekers—including Erich.

At fifteen he made a pilgrimage to the Self-Realization Fellowship center, on the cliffs overlooking the Pacific in Encinitas, California. The oceanside hermitage had been prophesied by Yogananda's guru, as he relates in his landmark book, *Autobiography of a Yogi*, and arriving there was a "definite pivotal point" for Erich. "The monks took me up to Yogananda's room and said, 'Look, you can still feel his vibe in here,' and there *was* something. And it was important to me."

At around the same time, Erich was being deeply affected by the writings of Jiddu

Practicing Cobra *(Bhujangasana)*

1. Lie on your abdomen with the forehead on the floor so the back of the neck is long. Place your palms alongside your chest with the wrists under the elbows, which point up to the ceiling. Curl your toes under and press the heels away until the kneecaps lift off the floor ❶. This is how active your legs should be in the yogic push-up pose, *Chaturanga* (Four-Limbed Staff).

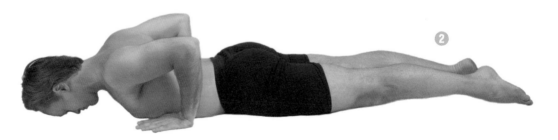

2. Keep your quadriceps engaged, so when you point your toes and spread all ten toenails into the floor, the knees remain lifted ❷. This is how your legs should feel in Upward-Facing Dog (*Urdhva Mukha Svanasana*), shown on p. 48. Pause here to notice the way in which your thighbones extend from the hip sockets. Are one or both of your legs rolling in or out? Work to redress such imbalances with the quality of your attention.

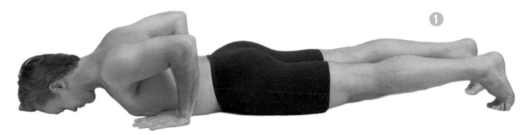

Krishnamurti, who had been arousing Western intellect since the Theosophical Society tapped him as a "world teacher" in the 1930s. "Somewhere in one of Krishnamurti's books it said that if you want to get your head together, it helps if you make your body sensitive," Erich says. "I was so enamored of anything he said, I took his advice."

Although he had already graduated from high school when he found out about Krishnamurti's secondary school in Brockwood Park, England, Erich decided he had to attend. His plan had been to go to college and study painting, but he figured he could do that the next year. His parents were reluctantly supportive, so Erich headed to Brockwood for an educational experience beyond what he could have envisioned.

"Seeing Krishnamurti walk down the hall or to have him look at you, you knew there was something more infinite looking through him looking at you; it wasn't just his ego-mind," Erich says. "And

to see someone living in a higher consciousness confirms that these teachings are real, that they're more than intellectual or fanciful thinking." The curriculum at Brockwood included hatha yoga classes, and since Erich connected so strongly with them, Krishnamurti recommended that he go to India to study with a teacher of his, T.K.V. Desikachar. "I thought, Okay, I'll do *that* for a year, and then I'll go to art school," Erich says. And so he left England for Madras.

It was 1972, and few Westerners had heard of Desikachar or his father, T. Krishnamacharya, who taught many of the yogis who developed today's prevalent yoga styles, including B.K.S. Iyengar, K. Pattabhi Jois, and Desikachar himself. Erich spent a year with Desikachar, learning the basics of what is now called Viniyoga. "It was so exciting to be there, and I saw Krishnamacharya almost every day, sitting there on the porch in a little wicker chair. I'd come up and salute him, '*Namaste*,' but

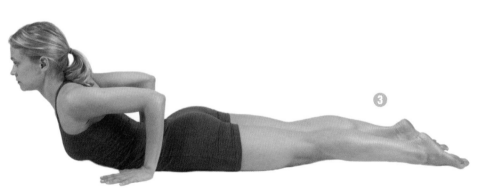

3. Maintaining active legs, slowly lift the head, neck, and chest off the floor ❸. Send your shoulders down toward your hips, and let your heart—not your chin and shoulders ❹—lead the way up. Try lifting your palms an inch off the floor to ensure that your back muscles are doing the work.

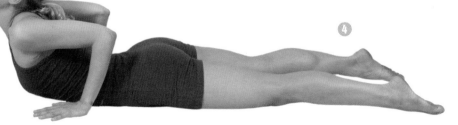

Cobra *(Bhujangasana)*

he never responded. And I thought that was so cool. I heard him say three things. One was 'Please lock your bicycle,' the second was 'Your teacher is not here today,' and the third was 'Yoga is not mechanical,' Erich recalls. "He looked beautiful, but his two front teeth were missing. That was the only thing."

When Erich left India, Brockwood chanced to be in need of a yoga teacher. "The perfect circumstance arose, and I was the yoga teacher suddenly." He spent the next five years teaching students and studying with nearby masters—B.K.S. Iyengar's senior European teacher, Dona Holleman, her student Mary Stewart—and with Iyengar himself, at a workshop he conducted in England. Then Erich journeyed to Rome to study with Vanda Scaravelli, another longtime Iyengar student, who evolved a radically feminine approach to asana.

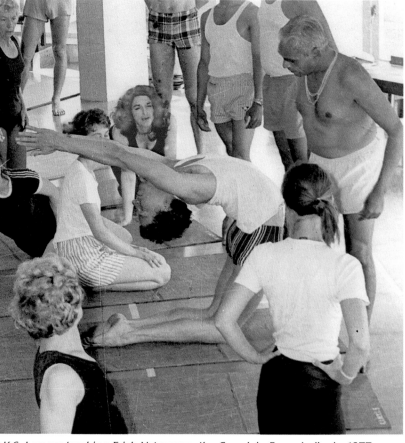

B.K.S. Iyengar teaching Erich Ustrasana, *the Camel, in Pune, India, in 1977.*

Scaravelli began studying yoga at age fifty and could drop into a backbend virtually until she died at ninety-one, in 1999. She was in her seventies when she greeted Erich at the train station in a red turban and little rubber flip-flops. "She was eccentric, eclectic, comfortable," he says. "I was really skinny and flexible, and I could do all this stuff. She would say, 'Don't be violent; take it easy.' She communicated the feeling that when you do yoga, let it be an expression of love." Scaravelli "got it" from her studies with Iyengar, Erich says, and she had the courage and passion to make her own pathway. In the summer of 1977 Erich returned to India—to Pune, this time—to "get" more Iyengar himself.

It was on Erich's return to Brockwood that a fellow Californian, yoga instructor Joel Kramer,

helped liberate the true teacher within Erich. What Kramer imparted to Erich was the means to become his own source of inspiration. "Now when I practice, I'm taking notes, and I'm learning—but not from me: I'm listening to the Infinite," he says. "That's what Iyengar does, and that's why he's been so creative."

Erich never did become a painter. His creativity manifested itself not in oils or acrylics but in teaching yoga, which his students would describe as no less an art. In 1994 one of his students, the actress Ali McGraw, made a video of Erich's teaching that heralded yoga's increasingly popular appeal. That popularization is something Erich applauds. "No matter the reason for someone's initial involvement, yoga works—and the more people do it, the more it will transform their lives."

Erich has not harked to the call of commercialism. There is no "Schiffmann Yoga" or

Schiffmann Yoga Studio. And despite all his experience with the greatest masters of our time, he maintains that the real initiations are internal. "It's not like you get certified by somebody else," he says. "The main deal is to listen inwardly, which is the essence of meditation.

"People often ask me, 'What kind of yoga do you teach?' And for the longest time I would say, 'Well, I've studied with so-and-so and so-and-so and so-and-so, and I've taken what I thought was the best from everybody and blended it with years of my own personal practice, and it comes out like this.' And one day someone said, 'Why don't you just call it Freedom Style?' So among my friends, we do. I like that because students and teachers who get into Freedom Style will not all look the same. How it comes through me is going to be different from how it comes through you. And yet we're both doing the same thing—listening inwardly and daring to do as the inner feeling says."

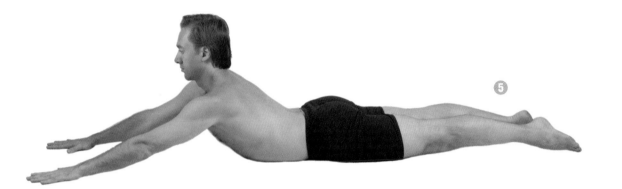

4. "Use your arms a little, then a little more," Erich suggests. "And once you get the structure, start letting the inner feeling guide you. Sometimes put your arms far forward ❺, sometimes put them back by your chest in the usual spot, and some of the time stretch them out sideways ❻. In that position you can lock your arms straight and have your shoulders down without having to be real deep in the pose. Occasionally, I like to cross my ankles with the legs straight and wiggle around like a seal ❼."

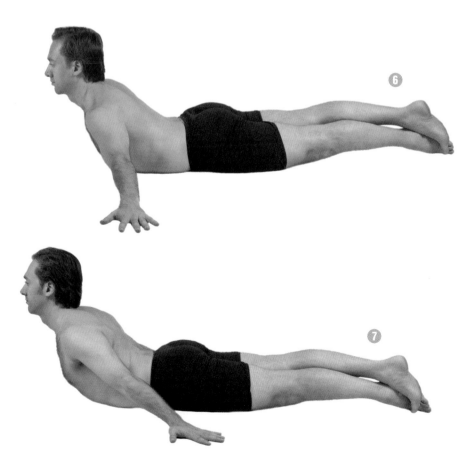

Cobra *(Bhujangasana)*

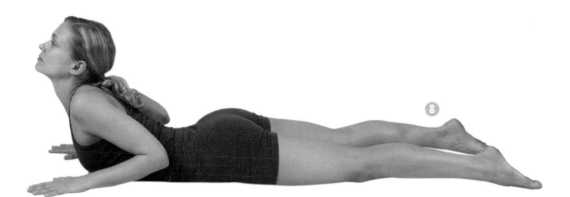

5. If you begin with poorly placed hands and legs in Cobra ❽, you will drag yourself into a poorly constructed Upward-Facing Dog (*Urdhva Mukha Svanasana*) ❾. So keep your palms and shoulders back and down and your quadriceps engaged ❿. Then as you draw your chest forward of your shoulders and your hips toward the heels of the hands, your knees and thighs will lift off the floor.

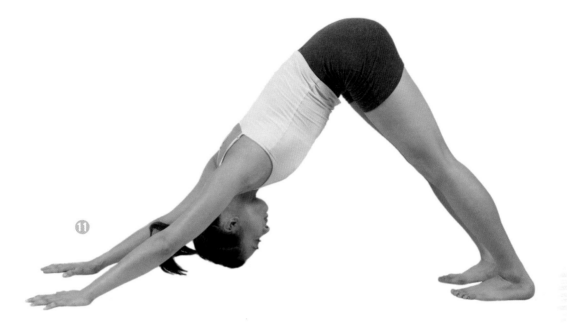

6. Mary Dunn recommends moving into a variation of Updog that teaches you what is necessary to avoid compressing the lower back in the pose. From Downward-Facing Dog ⑪, keep your toes tucked as you bring the legs down toward the floor and draw your chest between your arms ⑫. Then stretch your arms and legs, pressing the fronts and backs of your legs up to the ceiling. "Letting your legs come down first teaches you how to take in the tailbone," Mary says. "If you don't have your tailbone in first, the arms can overpower the chest, and it will go backward. And lifting the legs up too strongly initially will just lift the buttocks and displace the attention to the tailbone—and all of that will shorten the spine."

Mary Dunn

Downward-Facing Dog
(Adho Mukha Svanasana)

M **ary Dunn is a premier American teacher** in the tradition of the Indian yoga master B.K.S. Iyengar. Her longtime devotion to the study of asana under his precise tutelage led her to cofound Iyengar centers in San Francisco, San Diego, and New York. Yet it was another yoga pioneer who first drew Mary to the practice.

Mary was already off to college in 1960 when her mother, Mary Palmer, began taking yoga classes at their local YMCA in Ann Arbor, Michigan. Mrs. Palmer's passion for the practice was further fueled by the 1966 publication of B.K.S. Iyengar's *Light on Yoga*, now considered the bible of yoga asanas. Nearly as inspiring to her as the book itself was the foreword by the violinist Yehudi Menuhin, whose lyric praise of both the practice and of his teacher resonated strongly with her. A music lover and avid pianist, Mary's mother was in attendance when Menuhin played a concert in Ann Arbor in 1968. But yoga was what she spoke with him about after the performance. Menuhin encouraged her to go study with Iyengar in Pune, India. She did so, and by 1973 Mary Palmer had brought B.K.S. Iyengar to teach yoga at the Ann Arbor Y.

"My mother instilled in me that you don't have to be satisfied with an ordinary experience, because extraordinary experiences exist in the world, and you just have to avail yourself of them," Mary Dunn says. Mary herself obtained a master's degree in education, taught English for three years, moved to San Francisco with her husband, and gave birth to her first child before she found her way to a yoga class. And although she considered the experience interesting, it did not become extraordinary until she met Iyengar on his second U.S. teaching tour—arranged by her mother—in 1974.

"After a half hour I knew I'd found something absolutely fascinating, because it spoke to my physical awareness as nothing ever had," Mary says. "I was very stiff, but Guruji taught me how I could use my intelligence to gain entry into postures other people could do because they were limber. Every place he connected—the heels to the

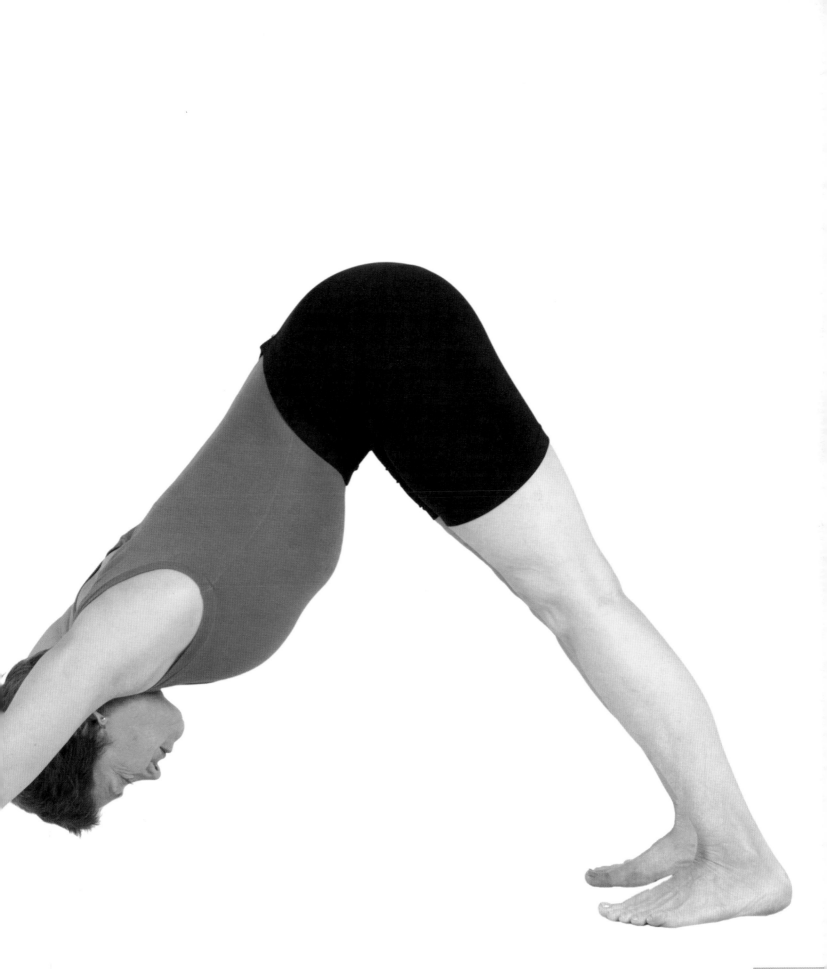

calves to the thighs or one leg to the other or one action to the other—was practical and brought change."

The change went far beyond anatomy. "He taught that the way you do asana reveals the way you do other things," Mary says. "He spoke about how the postures reveal your state of mind and about what you can do physically to bring about emotional repose. And I thought, This is intelligence used to survey, understand, and direct life on all kinds of levels."

Iyengar's teachings inspired yoga teachers in the San Francisco Bay area to continue studying his methodology. Mary became an ever more keen student and in 1976 made her first trip to Pune with her mother. Her father came to help her husband take care of their two girls. If Mary's mother was avant-garde, the men in her family

THE YOGA OF THE POSE: "It is a wonderful posture to begin practice with because it takes me to the way I access the beauty of asana—which is going from the limbs, the *karmendriyas*, to the center of the body. The pose uses all four limbs equally; that's why it's named after our favorite four-limbed companion. It teaches about the joints in those limbs, so the limbs can be used in the most effective way to open us to the experience of our essence. It opens us to our breath, to the spine, to the way the limbs can connect us into all the muscles of the body. When you stretch your arms, the extension takes you into the shoulder blades and the postural muscles that cover the trunk. It gives you access to places that are hard to access without the connection from the limbs.

"The posture is marvelous also in that having the head down takes you into the essence of *pratyahara* (p. 56), because it is a departure from our usual way of looking at and listening to the world at eye and ear level. It's a partial inversion, too, which changes the physiological balance of the body."

HOW STUDENTS COMMONLY MISS IT: "By falling into what's easy and by not knowing how to adjust for restriction. Either prevents us from establishing intelligent connection with the limbs and from taking advantage of our limbs' ability to open the rest of the body.

"Flexibility can keep us from exploring the fineness of doing. And severely restricted practitioners—people with very tight hamstrings and shoulders or an exaggerated thoracic curve—may never get to know the pose at all without proper instruction."

HOW TO MAKE SURE YOU CONNECT: "Use your arms and legs in a balanced, intelligent way to access openness of the spine, freedom of the breath, and the quietness of mental and emotional stability. Stretch the elbows and knees well, and concentrate on and develop how the limbs both support and open the body. Also concentrate on discovering the relationship of the center body to the support. Use the pose to refine and expand the understanding of the extension of the spine that comes from that.

"Extend from the hands through the arms through the side body all the way up to the buttock bones. Then develop that same awareness in the legs. Students with limited hamstring flexibility should begin with the heels neither actively lifted nor pressing down so they can extend through the knees first. Once you extend the lower leg away from the upper leg, stretch equally down into heels and up into thighs. You have to learn how to do both. Then coordinate that action with the rhythm of how you stretch through the hands and arms and side body.

"As you get to know the pose you're drawn into a better understanding of the things you knew about it. The details and techniques of it become integrated, and the whole experience of being there over time starts to extend till you learn to take away tension. You end up with a pose that's extended and full of action without tension—which allows you to examine all the psychological ramifications of being rather than doing that can only happen when a pose is mature."

were forward thinking as well. Mary's husband buttressed her growth as a yoga teacher, and her father "was probably one of the first people in the United States doing Sun Salutations," Mary says. Mr. Palmer was the only American member of his university's Hindustani Club in the 1920s. "He wasn't a Hindu, but he had a lot of Indian friends," Mary explains. "And one of them taught him *Surya Namaskar.*" Mary, it seems, was a destined force in American yoga.

After returning from her first three-week intensive with Iyengar, Mary began filling in for her teacher in San Francisco. Eventually Mary helped establish the teacher-training program that in 1978 became the San Francisco Iyengar Yoga Institute. A year later, when she and her husband moved to San Diego, she launched the Iyengar center there. She was also a teacher at the Los Angeles institute, where she traveled regularly to train teachers. And when she and her family relocated to New York, she cofounded the Iyengar Yoga Association of New York, which established the New York institute in 1993.

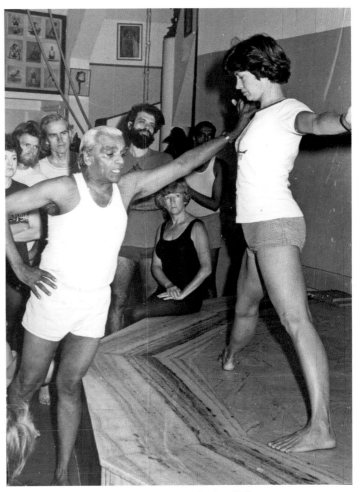

Mary with B.K.S. Iyengar in Pune, India, in 1978.

Mary has never been drawn to any other style of yoga. "There's so much to pursue in this practice that I don't feel limited in any way," she says. "Iyengar Yoga is a huge umbrella. For students who get great joy from cultivating vitality, there are ways of practicing that are as active and challenging as Astanga Yoga. The *vinyasa* practices I learned from Guruji back in the '70s started with Sun Salutations. Then he would put in almost any pose in the book. It wasn't 'Get this one form first and then the second and then the third'; it was freer than that.

"For people who are wise but limited physically, I can teach from the wisdom of yoga to their wisdom and appreciation of life," Mary says. "And I can teach to people who are intellectual and to people who are more into the feeling that yoga

brings. So this particular umbrella suits me because it has so many aspects.

"People have incorrectly pigeonholed Iyengar Yoga into 'alignment, technique, props' rather than 'learning, experiencing, integrating'—which I think are the real words," Mary says. That image may prevail because so many Iyengar teachers imitate their guru's brilliance without approaching it, as is the case in any movement sparked by one person's genius. But Mary also points to the fact that "people have to have their own brand on something. This is life; I'm not being critical. But there is no question that Iyengar has been the source of what many people in all styles teach from. Then they spread off because they want to have a movement based on themselves; they don't want to be the disciple."

Downward-Facing Dog *(Adho Mukha Svanasana)*

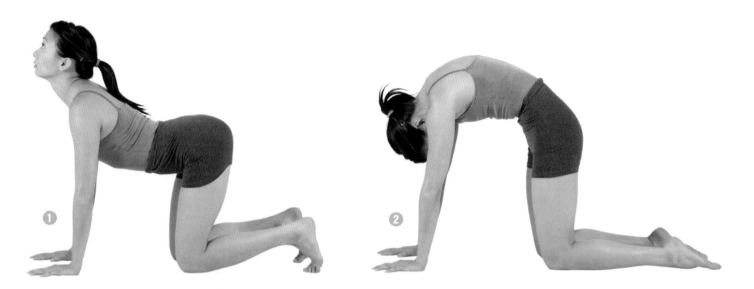

Practicing Downward-Facing Dog *(Adho Mukha Svanasana)*

1. A nice way to warm the spine for Down Dog is the sequence generally referred to as Cat/Cow. Come to your hands and knees with your wrists directly below your shoulders and knees right under your hips ❶. On an inhale curl the toes under, lift the tailbone, drop the belly, open the chest, and look up. As you exhale, point your feet and press the shins and tops of feet down as you round the spine and push the middle of the back to the ceiling ❷. (As you draw your navel toward your spine here, this is a good place to begin to understand *uddiyana bandha* [p. 29].) Repeat this sequence, marrying breath with movement.

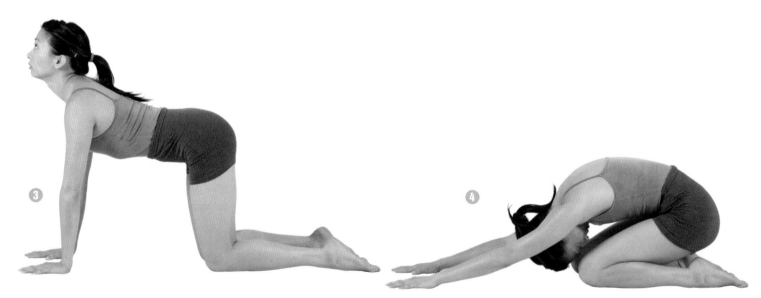

2. Also try *Chakravakasana*, Viniyoga's more circumspect version of the pose. As you inhale, lift the sternum, keeping the low back relatively flat ❸. On one slow exhalation, draw the navel toward the spine and slowly lengthen both sitting bones back toward your heels ❹. (Try humming your exhalation and see how that deepens the work.) Come down progressively lower on each exhale, bringing the chest toward the thighs before the buttocks reach the heels.

3. Teach yourself how the Down Dog torso should feel by doing what Erich Schiffmann calls Half Dog ⑤. From hands-and-knees position keep your hips over your knees and walk the arms forward till your forehead rests on the floor or a block, if you need one. Activate the hands and forearms so the elbows stay lifted. Also observe how pressing into the thumb and index finger ball joints allows the shoulders to roll to the outer edges of the room while the forearms seek each other out—another key to proper use of the limbs.

⑤

4. From the Half Dog take an easy twist by lowering your right shoulder onto the floor, turning your head left, and gazing up beyond your left shoulder ⑥. This is a lovely pose in which to experience *sukha*, the comfortable quality each asana is designed to comprise. Feel it here where it's easy, so you can replicate it when it's not.

⑥

Mary, on the other hand, is the quintessential American disciple, and she remains clear about why that is. "Mr. Iyengar says to start with asana because that's where we live. Most of us are not going to move step by step through the eight-limbed path (p. 56) because only saints get all the *yamas* right before they go on. Each limb is something we work on and get insight on all the time. We practice *dhyana, pratyahara*, all of those other things *in the venue*—that's how we experience life, in the venue of asana. It's not about how straight we stand, but about how much we're in touch with ourselves. All of this deals with philosophy. For him it is all one subject."

If Iyengar Yoga is considered the "technique one," Mary says, it is because technique promotes concentration, one of the higher limbs. "It's the alignment with concentration, the extension and finding the point of concentration, then combining that with another point of concentration and finding the places where those two points blend that allows us to experience spreading of the mind," she says. "It's one thing to say, 'Now we're going to spread the mind.' It's another thing to experience it. You can say, 'Close your eyes and spread your mind,' and sometimes that works for people and other times they wonder, Well, am I doing it? But with something as clear as the Iyengar method, you know you've been somewhere else. You know it."

ASTANGA: THE EIGHT-LIMBED PATH

By 200 A.D., a writer named Patanjali had codified the already ancient philosophy of yoga in a text called the *Yoga Sutras.* Theretofore passed on orally, his 196 sutras, or aphorisms, delineate how to arrive at the state of yoga, which he defined as control of the fluctuations of the mind. If, as Richard Miller says, yoga is a "series of experiments designed to help you inquire into who you are and what the nature of reality is," *astanga yoga,* the eight-limbed path, described in the *Sutras'* second chapter, is the handbook.

1. Restraints (Yamas)
    nonviolence *(ahimsa)*
    not lying *(satya)*
    not stealing *(asteya)*
    not lusting *(bramacharya)*
    not possessing *(aparigraha)*
2. Observances (Niyamas)
    cleanliness *(saucha)*
    contentment *(santosha)*
    discipline *(tapas)*
    Self-study *(svadhyaya)*
    surrender to the highest *(Isvara pranidhana)*
3. Postures (Asana)
4. Breath expansion (Pranayama)
5. Sense withdrawal (Pratyahara)
6. Concentration (Dharana)
7. Meditation (Dhyana)
8. Absorption in Supreme Consciousness (Samadhi)

People have been interpreting the *Sutras* since they were written, and the women and men in this book continue the tradition. Nischala Joy Devi believes that the text has been broadly misconstrued, from the concept of *brahmacharya*—"which means not celibacy, but moderation in everything we do so that we can begin to feel and see God"—to the definition of yoga mentioned above. "Yoga is not about control," she says. "It is about union, the bringing together of all the aspects of ourselves so that we can feel the spirit in the heart."

Her colleagues have made their own conclusions. "We can look at the *Sutras* as a progressive teaching or as a direct teaching that's pointing right to our true nature," Richard Miller says. "So one could look at yoga as 'doing'—we're trying to learn to *be* stillness—or that yoga is understanding that we *are* stillness." That per-

spective can be applied to all the limbs, he says. "Take *satya:* Is Patanjali using the word saying 'Be truthful,' or 'your true nature is truthfulness'? I think he uses it in both ways."

Tim Miller agrees. "The *yamas* and *niyamas* are not necessarily rules you need to follow to achieve the state of yoga, but are more an outgrowth of your immersion in the state of yoga. Asana practice is a prerequisite for *pranayama,* which is a prerequisite for meditation; but asana is also a foundation for cultivating a sense of your place in the world. You experience union on the physical level and then build on that sense of union."

"Asana is Mental Training 101," Beryl Bender Birch says. "You're training the mind for *dharana.* Through *mula bandha, uddiyana bandha, ujjayi* breathing, *drishti*— all these mindfulness techniques that accompany my particular tradition—you're learning to focus on one thing without distraction or interruption. It's a process of moving from the most gross to the most subtle."

Patricia Sullivan likes the flexibility in what initially can seem like a rigid prescription for bliss, as *samadhi* is sometimes defined. "One of the things I appreciate is that Patanjali lists the many different ways there are to calm the mind and see our true nature," she says. "You can do it through dreams, through chanting Om, through the breath, through devotion to God—whatever way appeals to you, because that's the way you can be devoted to."

That level of participation is key to the practice of *pratyahara,* Krishna Kaur says. "Yogi Bhajan translated *pratyahara* as synchronization as opposed to sense control: to be totally in harmony with the whole universal experience so no one sense is more dominant than the other. If you withdraw into 'No senses, no senses! No senses are being expressed or dealt with here!' you have misperception, *avidya.* If you can harmonize and equalize all sensations, then you have experienced *pratyahara.*"

"The whole thrust of the *Yoga Sutras* is that what is arising is sacred, and so you can pay exquisitely close attention to it," Richard Freeman notes. "Right now is a worthy object of your meditation."

Dharma Mittra offers a similarly unequivocal definition of the final limb, *samadhi.* "When you are ready to enter the temple, the sacred chamber of your heart, and see reality, it's like that commercial for the Roach Motel," he says. "You check in, and you never check out." When he laughs, something tells you he might be there.

5. To move into Downward-Facing Dog (*Adho Mukha Svanasana*), lift your hips up and back and straighten the legs until you are shaped like an inverted V, with your tailbone at its pinnacle ❼. If you have tight shoulders and hamstrings, you may look more like a Q ❽. To experience the elongated spine that makes Down Dog what Mary Dunn calls a "marvelous pose," bend your knees till your ribs move toward your thighs and sling your hips up and back ❾.

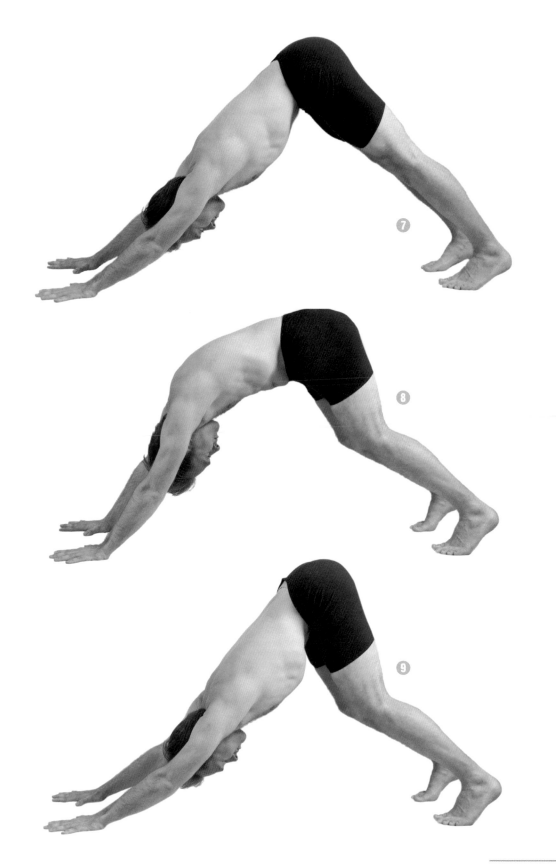

Downward-Facing Dog *(Adho Mukha Svanasana)*

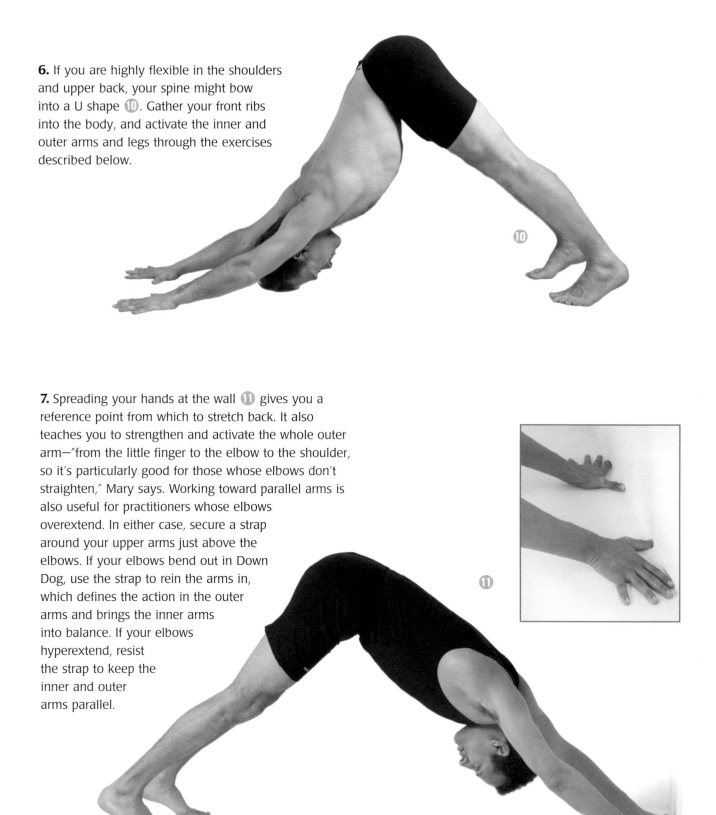

6. If you are highly flexible in the shoulders and upper back, your spine might bow into a U shape ⑩. Gather your front ribs into the body, and activate the inner and outer arms and legs through the exercises described below.

7. Spreading your hands at the wall ⑪ gives you a reference point from which to stretch back. It also teaches you to strengthen and activate the whole outer arm—"from the little finger to the elbow to the shoulder, so it's particularly good for those whose elbows don't straighten," Mary says. Working toward parallel arms is also useful for practitioners whose elbows overextend. In either case, secure a strap around your upper arms just above the elbows. If your elbows bend out in Down Dog, use the strap to rein the arms in, which defines the action in the outer arms and brings the inner arms into balance. If your elbows hyperextend, resist the strap to keep the inner and outer arms parallel.

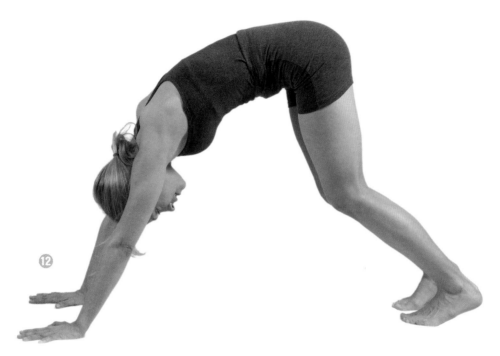

8. If you do not connect through the hands and feet, you cannot lengthen your spine away from the floor ⑫. Use your hands as if you were a tree frog climbing a tree. Spread the fingers evenly with the middle finger facing forward and press down on the base of all three knuckles of each finger.

Energize the legs and feet as much as the arms and hands. Open the backs of the knees in the way Mary suggests if you are restricted in hamstring flexibility. If your heels come easily to the floor and you have a tendency to hyperextend the backs of your knees, use this tip from John Friend: Actively and simultaneously press your shinbones forward and your thighbones back to reteach yourself how to stretch the hamstrings beneficially.

Learn to use the limbs—and your mind—evenly by introducing unevenness into the situation ⑬. Lift one leg straight up behind you, keeping the hips and shoulders level and both sides of the waist long. Hold for five breaths and repeat on the other side.

Tim Miller

Warrior One
(Virabhadrasana I)

As he has for nearly a quarter century, Tim Miller quietly runs the Ashtanga Yoga Center in Encinitas, California, the school he came to and then inherited from two of the earliest American practitioners of the discipline. Tim himself was the first Westerner ever certified by the Astanga Yoga guru K. Pattabhi Jois—"probably because I'm the first one who asked," he demurs. Yet despite unquestionable dedication to and primacy in this highly structured method of practice, Tim remains steadfastly nonrigid about it all.

"I like to think yoga continues to evolve as we do," he says. "It's not something invented five thousand years ago that we have to endlessly repeat in this traditional fashion. I have great respect for the tradition, which gives you a good sense of what a practice should consist of—that it has a definite beginning, middle, and end, and that it's sequenced so each part prepares you for the next. But it's like learning to play music: Once you get a firm grasp of the scales, at some point you're going to want to create something more you."

Tim's introduction to the practice of yoga came from a book, Swami Satchidananda's *Integral Yoga Hatha.* A briefly incarcerated friend had gotten the book from another short-termer at the county lockup, and on his release, he passed it on to Tim. At the time, Tim was studying psychology and Eastern philosophy at the University of California at Riverside. He began teaching himself yoga, and when he moved to Encinitas to work in a psychiatric hospital, he took the book with him. It came in handy.

"Based on my very limited experience of yoga I actually started teaching it to psychiatric patients," Tim says. "I taught a mishmash of stuff I had gleaned from Swami Satchidananda's book and also from the famous stretching book by Bob Anderson. They weren't a very discriminating audience, so they thought I was great."

Fortunately, Tim says, a yoga center opened half a block from where he was living. What was being taught there was Astanga Yoga. "The first class I took blew my mind. It felt like I found what I had been looking for my whole life. That was it for me." Nine months later he took class with Pattabhi Jois, right there in Encinitas, which Tim calls the American birthplace for this practice. The southern California beach town was home to David Williams and Nancy Gilgoff, who first imported the discipline and the master—in

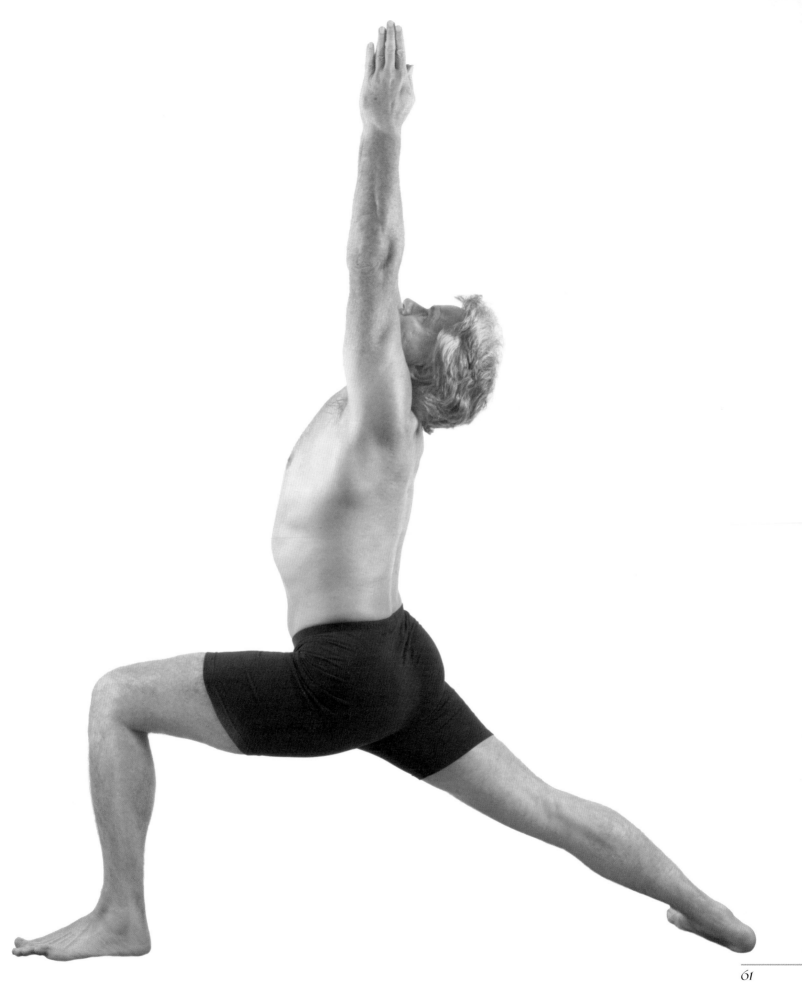

Warrior One *(Virabhadrasana I)*

THE YOGA OF THE POSE: "The sense of sacred geometry. When you find that, there's just a rightness to the pose that's also very appealing aesthetically. The front thighbone is parallel to the floor, the torso and arms are absolutely perpendicular, the plane of the face points directly up. External alignment is a manifestation of internal clarity or a sense of paying attention to the task at hand. And out of that stability you can begin to go deeper."

HOW STUDENTS COMMONLY MISS IT: "By not going deep enough. Things happen when you go deeper into the pose that just don't if you hang above it all. A lot of people complain about having stiff hips, and when you watch the way they do their warrior poses, they do them at such a shallow level they don't even get into the hips very much.

"Another common thing is for people with hyperflexible backs to drop into the lumbar spine till it looks like a backbend. The articulation or extension of the spine needs to begin from the coccyx. And some people take the head back too far, but more often they don't take it back far enough."

HOW TO MAKE SURE YOU CONNECT: "Put forth some effort. If you don't, you don't make progress. On a physical level the strongly rooted back leg is the force that drives the pelvis forward and allows you to go deeper into the front leg. Work to get the front femur bone parallel to the floor, but if the back foot lifts, you lose the foundation, so don't go beyond the point where you begin to lose the outer edge of the foot.

"As you deepen the work, cultivate a sense of detachment so that you're no longer the show, you're just watching the show: you are what Patanjali calls the *drashtu*. That's the inherent irony of yoga—that we're working hard to experience something that's already present. So be the witness, not the victim. Watch the show."

Practicing Warrior One *(Virabhadrasana I)*

1. From Downward-Facing Dog ❶ step one foot forward between your hands so that your toenails and fingernails are in one horizontal line. (Draw the foot forward with your hand if it falls short.) Bend your front knee to a 90-degree angle and lower your back heel to the floor. When learning the pose, it can be helpful to drop your head and look between your legs ❷ to see that the back foot is angled in with its outer edge pressed into the floor. Align your back heel with your front heel, and maintain your foundation well as you circle your arms out and up and join the palms overhead in a prayer ❸.

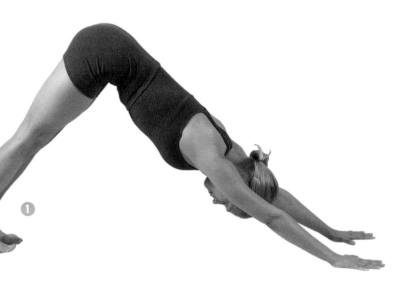

1975 and next in 1978, when Tim was on hand to meet him. "I just happened to be in the right place at the right time," he says.

Tim continued to study with his teacher whenever he could, in the States and over some eleven trips to India. "The first trip convinced me that my dharma was to be a yoga teacher. So I thought that to have his blessing was important." With his high degree of dedication and flexibility, Tim had become proficient at Astanga Yoga's first three series before he went to Pattabhi Jois's school in Mysore. So with youthful aplomb, at the end of his visit he asked for and was granted formal certification to teach the method.

Does his early experience teaching psychiatric patients have any bearing on how he instructs the healthy, athletic types that comprise a typical Astanga Yoga class? "Yes, well, sometimes the world seems like one big mental hospital," Tim says. "But one thing that has always amazed me is the plasticity of the human mind, how shapeable it is and how susceptible to all the vagaries of experience. Traditionally yoga has been approached from the spiritual perspective and more recently, in this country, from the physical perspective. But to me the most interesting part is the psychological. I like to see the kind of changes it works on people. It affects them deeply.

"With psychiatric patients there was no pretense; they were in trouble. And yoga was a tool that was helpful. Afterward you could see in their faces some sense of clarity and appreciation for being alive." But in general, "people tend to do their yoga practice the way they live their lives. It becomes a reflection of the personality. Students whose faces are screwed up in pain are not having a good time. You have to remind them where they are—in this wonderful country, immersed in the practice of Self-realization."

For Tim the stricture of the form of Astanga Yoga continues to expand as a practice and as a teaching. In the mid-1980s, he began exploring what he calls *Surya Namaskar C*, a sort of "yoga

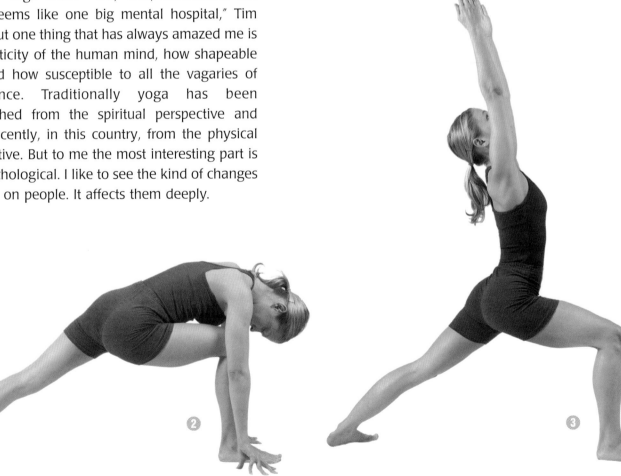

Warrior One *(Virabhadrasana I)*

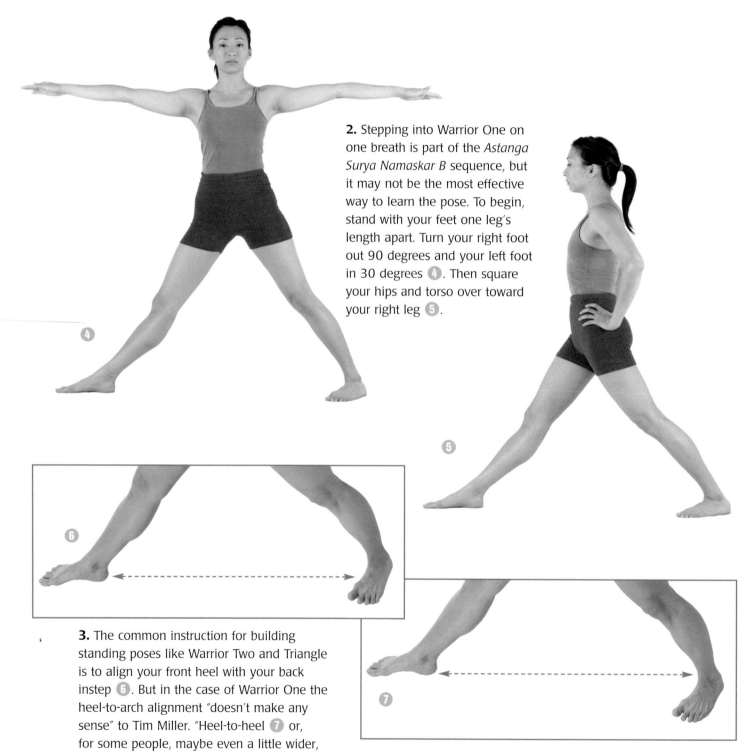

2. Stepping into Warrior One on one breath is part of the *Astanga Surya Namaskar B* sequence, but it may not be the most effective way to learn the pose. To begin, stand with your feet one leg's length apart. Turn your right foot out 90 degrees and your left foot in 30 degrees ❹. Then square your hips and torso over toward your right leg ❺.

3. The common instruction for building standing poses like Warrior Two and Triangle is to align your front heel with your back instep ❻. But in the case of Warrior One the heel-to-arch alignment "doesn't make any sense" to Tim Miller. "Heel-to-heel ❼ or, for some people, maybe even a little wider, seems to accommodate the width of hips and movement of sacrum better, and it's easier to get the back hip to rotate forward and to get the twisting motion of the torso." Try it both ways to see what "gives better action," Tim recommends.

jazz" rooted in a class he took from a fellow teacher named Roger Cole. "Roger is a pretty traditional Iyengar teacher, but the class he taught that day was called 'vinyasa.' He'd take standing poses with common themes, common actions, and link them all together. I thought, This is kind of cool. I like this. But it didn't have the sense of flow I'm used to from Astanga Yoga. So I decided I would use this idea and try to add smoothness through integrating breath and movement, using *Chaturanga* and Downward Dogs to add fluidity to it all. I started playing with that, a sort of endless improvisation with each position in the Sun Salutation as a foundation to launch into another sequence.

"In the early 1990s some of the up-and-coming young yoga stars would take my workshops at Yoga Works in Santa Monica. When I was playing around with *Surya Namaskar C*, they were in there learning those sequences. So perhaps I planted some kind of seed in their mind for this 'vinyasa flow' style. I had found that doing the same practice in the same sequence day after day gets a little monotonous, so once or twice a week I do something more improvisational, but using Astanga principles. Sequencing works only if it goes somewhere. In some *vinyasa* flow classes, it's a lot of work and sweat and huffin' and puffin', but

WARRIOR UNKNOTTED
Tim Miller recalls his teacher's comment that *Virabhadrasana I* addresses the *granthis,* or knots, that block the pathway of rising energy in the body. "If you can be focused on where your body is located in space, you're working toward releasing the *brahma granthi*, the creator's knot, there at the sacrum. By maintaining good *ujjayi* breath (p. 18), which is always going to be apparent by the quality of the sound, you're creating a sense of spaciousness around the heart, the *vishnu granthi*. And amid all this you maintain equanimity of mind through the one-pointed gaze, the *anatara drishti*, gazing into the infinite, that sense of timelessness and goallessness, which relates to the *siva granthi*, between the eyebrows. So if you get all three of those things working— what in Astanga Yoga is called the *tristhana*— they will keep you in the present moment."

there's no real sense of direction to it."

The direction of Tim's practice has grown sharper and sweeter, something he says is typical among longtime adherents of the hard practice of Astanga Yoga. "Yoga is fifty percent trying to make it happen and fifty percent allowing it to happen. It's a folly of youth to make it ninety percent effort and ten percent surrender. But if you stick around a while, you get better at the latter. I find with age I can't make it happen like I used to, so I am more conscious of allowing things to happen by softening and paying attention."

The birth of Tim's daughter brought what he considers a highly advanced variation to his practice: long walks on the beach "holding her in her little carrier, heart to heart. The ability to be at one with the object of your attention—that's what meditation is for me."

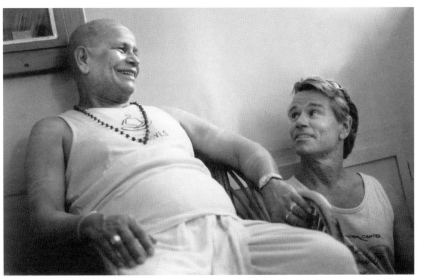
Tim with Sri K. Pattabhi Jois in Mysore, India, in 1999.

4. A good way to understand Warrior One is to move into and out of it "dynamically," as the Viniyoga tradition phrases it. (Tim Miller teaches beginning Warriors this way, too.) Start with your arms alongside your body and your legs straight ⑧. Inhale, press your palms overhead in a prayer, and look up ⑨. As you exhale, bend your front knee and descend into the pose while keeping the torso, palms, and gaze lifted ⑩. Inhale and straighten the front leg again ⑪, then exhale and release your arms alongside your body ⑫. Repeat several times on each side until you understand how the breath guides you into the pose.

5. Use muscle and awareness to keep the knee and thigh from rolling in or out, and guard against collapsing into the pose. If your front knee extends past your ankle, you need a wider stance. "When people with hyperflexible backs do the pose, they look like they're doing a backbend," Tim notes ⑬. "The articulation or extension of the spine needs to begin from the coccyx. *Mula bandha* articulates the coccyx and *uddiyhana bandha* articulates the sacrum and lumbar spine."

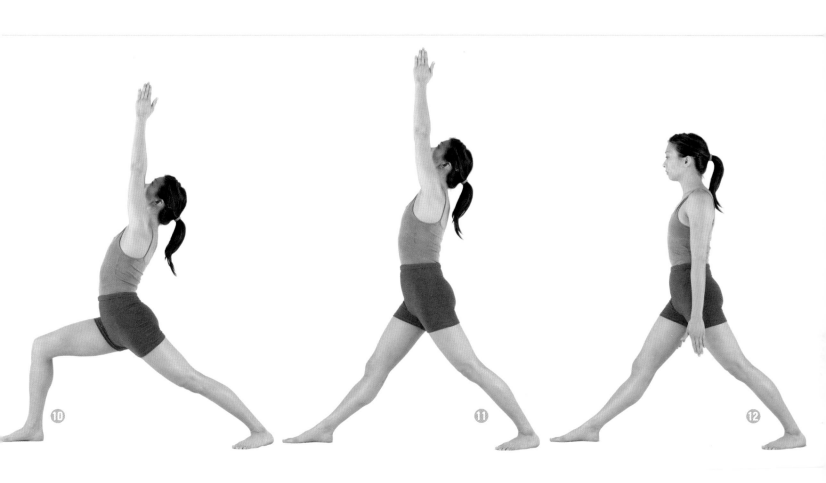

6. Viniyoga's gently integrative take on the pose teaches the importance of the back leg in relation to opening across the chest ⑭. It is especially useful for students with tight hips and an excessively curved thoracic spine. Take a narrower stance of about three feet. Bend your elbows and open your arms out and back, bringing the chest forward of the shoulders without overarching the low back. Root your tailbone through the outer edge of your back foot. As you breathe, lift and expand into your chest and across your collarbones.

Krishna Kaur
Kundalini Frog

Krishna Kaur has taught Kundalini Yoga in this country for the past thirty-three years. She heads up the International Association of Black Yoga Teachers and is the founder of Yoga for Youth, a nonprofit organization that sends yoga teachers into prisons and community centers nationwide. In a not-so-distant past life Krishna starred in Broadway musicals—under a name she declines to reveal. But if her comportment now is traditionally Indian, her implementation of yoga is radically American.

Krishna opened the first yoga center in South Central Los Angeles in 1971. It took a while to catch on. "People were asking, 'What is *that*? Is that something you eat?'" she says. "And I would talk to them about yoga, and they'd say, 'Well, it sounds fine, but how is it going to help me when I've got to put food on the table? When they're trying to cut off my lights? When the cops are down there beating everybody up for no reason at all?' I had to listen deeply in order to speak to that part that was reached when my teacher spoke to me. I couldn't say it the way he said it to me. I tried, but they didn't get it that way."

Krishna "got it" herself through an apparently circuitous route. In 1968, at the height of her early success as a dancer and actress in New York, she abandoned those endeavors, which "suddenly just didn't seem important," she says, and embarked on a quest to find out what was. "It was during the civil rights activities, and I thought, There's got to be something more I can do for my people than entertain them for two and a half hours at night."

Krishna had already begun investigating the ancient African religion Yoruba, which black Americans were then beginning to reclaim, when she found herself drawn to a slim volume on a bookstore shelf called *Science of Breath* by Yogi Ramacharaka. "For some reason I bought it and took it home," she says. "And within a week I was meditating, working with the breath, and had become a vegetarian." Her Yoruba mentor was not impressed. "Yoga is for the Indians," he told her. "If you want to find what's for you, you've got to go to Africa."

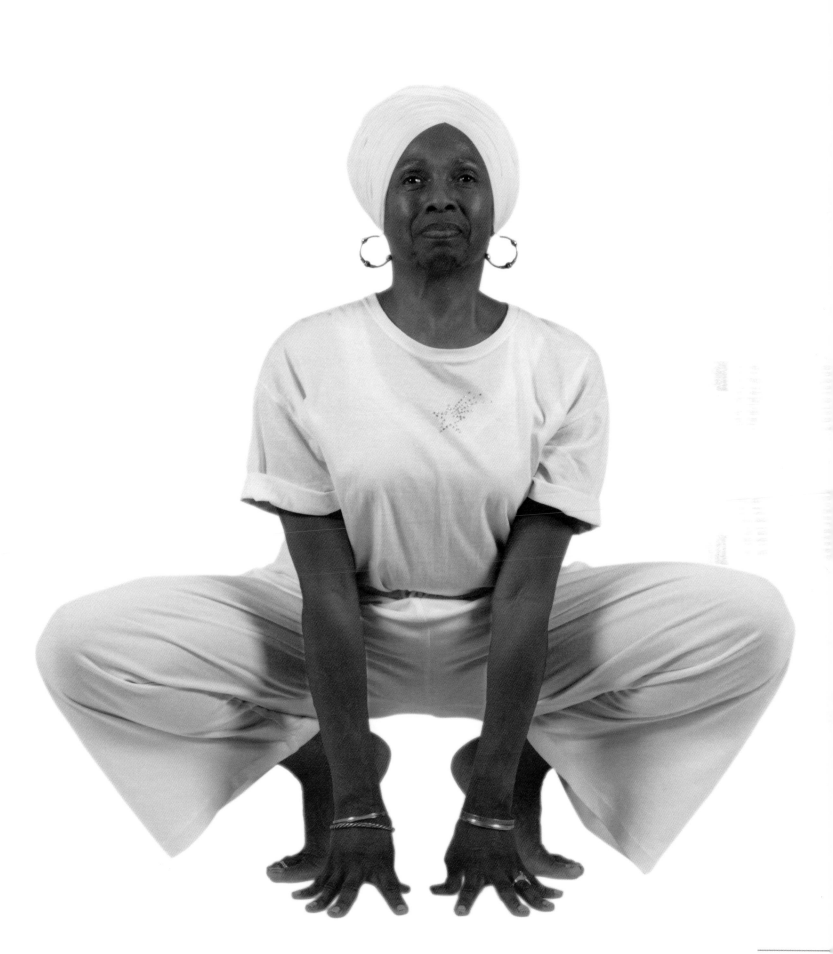

And so she did. But what took root during her year of travel was an increasing passion for yoga, which seemed intent on finding her. "The Yoruba religion was beautiful, but as I learned more about it, I realized it was not my faith," she says. "And whenever confusion set in, I'd invariably find myself in the house of someone who'd happen to have a book on yoga just sitting there. I'd gulp it down, and it would totally center and focus me." When she left Africa and headed back to the States, Krishna had no idea what she would do next, only that it would somehow involve yoga.

She attended her first yoga class at a June 1970 event in Boulder, Colorado, called the Holy Man Jam. "Swami Satchidananda, Yogi Bhajan—all these spiritual teachers were outside doing yoga and meditation with thousands of young people, and I just jumped in, and it felt so good," she says. "I went back for another class the very next night, and the teacher was this black guy named Salome—which reversed in my mind the earlier advice of my mentor. I gave myself permission to just close my eyes and do the practice, and it was wonderful."

The practice was Kundalini Yoga, which harnesses strong, often continuous, breathing techniques in combination with postures, meditation, and chanting to unlock the divine energy said to reside at the base of the spine. Yogi Bhajan brought the discipline to this country and in 1969 established 3HO, the Happy, Healthy, Holy Organization, and eventually a teacher training program, in which Krishna is an active participant.

"Yogi Bhajan came with a different technique that hadn't been passed on as openly as hatha yoga," she says. "And he ran into quite a bit of resistance from India—that he was sharing all these secret meditations and practices that they felt could not be appreciated by Americans." They were certainly appreciated by Krishna. "I took

THE YOGA OF THE POSE: "It's the whole choreography of movement and posture and breath, which comes together in this stew of overall benefits. The repetitive motion driven by inhales and exhales allows for a tremendous amount of lung expansion while it relieves the body of toxins. And the pace of the movements and breath is rapid because that forces the energy through the spine, up the channels of *ida* and *pingala*. That's a very important part of Kundalini Yoga—moving the energy from one place to another. And that's why the sequence is done the way it is, because it actually takes you from A to B.

"Twenty-six repetitions are good, but the optimal number is 108. When you repeatedly stand and squat in Frog pose, you exert pressure on the fleshy part of the big toe, where there's a meridian point that connects to the pituitary gland. So the pose stimulates pituitary gland secretion while it opens the hips and relaxes the sacrum."

HOW STUDENTS COMMONLY MISS IT: "By thinking, I can't. By never challenging themselves, because their indoctrination is more toward staying where it's comfortable than pushing up against perceived limitations. If you're thinking you can't, you've just wiped yourself out. You have no energy."

HOW TO MAKE SURE YOU CONNECT: "Go, 'Yeeeeessss!' Turn no into yes. Realize the power of your own mind, your own projection. If you say, 'Yes, yes,' and approach it like that, then you can sustain it. Think, This is not all of me; there's more of me left. If you want to excel in anything, you're going to have to experience the sensation of stretch. And that's what Kundalini offers, because it definitely can give you that pushing sensation. I've heard it described as a very easy style of yoga, and I just put my hand over my mouth and snicker. I think, Okay."

some hatha yoga classes afterward, and I liked the stretch and the open feeling. But I found that the Kundalini challenged me more and worked through any little resistances I had."

Krishna went to study with Yogi Bhajan a few months later in Phoenix, where he was conducting a ten-day course in White Tantra Yoga. Contrary to popular misconception, White Tantra does not involve sex, but explores the polarities of male and female energy through meditation, breath, and chanting practices. "The idea is to heal subconscious imbalances that interfere with the ability to elevate consciousness," Krishna says. And beyond the threshold of the physical challenges that often accompany such a concentrated course of intense practice, she experienced a reservoir of joy, peace, and deep meditation. "It was unbelievable," she says. "It changed everything."

Yogi Bhajan invited a group of students to accompany him to India shortly thereafter, and

Krishna signed on. "India looked like Africa, smelled like Africa, sounded like Africa," she says, and she spent her time in constant meditation and practice with the Kundalini Yoga master. Back in America, she moved into Yogi Bhajan's ashram in Los Angeles, where she remained for the next seven years. But the serenity she had enjoyed with her guru in India was not to be repeated in the City of Angels.

"He pushed me to go out to teach right away," Krishna recalls. "And in my mind I was screaming, No, no, no, I don't know anything! Don't make me do this! He said, 'You have to find a way to reach your people.' And I thought, My people? Who are my people? Everybody's my people. After returning from Africa and studying yoga in the U.S., I felt I didn't belong to any country, that the universe is my country. But he insisted I give it a try, and that's one of the things I honor in him the most. Because he did not let me get away with staying in my

Practicing Kundalini Frog

1. Squat deeply with your knees and toes open wide and your heels together and off the floor ❶. Place your fingertips on the floor about six inches in front of your feet. As you inhale, straighten your legs and draw your head toward your knees ❷, and as you exhale, lower back down to the squat, keeping your heels lifted and your spine long. To gain the benefits of this classic Kundalini sequence, Krishna Kaur recommends twenty-six repetitions fueled by strong inhalations and exhalations through the nose.

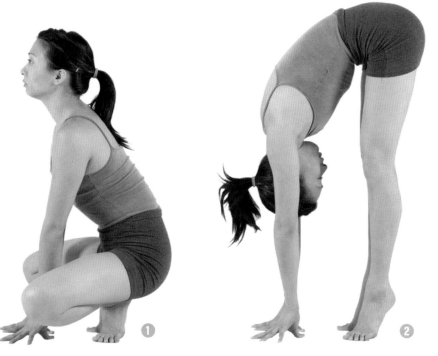

comfort zone—which is what a teacher is for."

Before long Krishna was teaching eighteen classes a week, had opened the Kundalini Yoga Drug Rehabilitation and Awareness Center (now called Tenth Gate), and was part of the South Central Los Angeles Planning Council, which tried to solve the issues of gang violence. She recalls spending a whole week teaching yoga classes in a high school gymnasium—"all day long, every gym class that came through," she says. "We had maybe two hundred kids sitting there, doing postures and breathing and meditating."

Krishna's work today continues to focus on young people, in schools and in prisons. "The idea is to try and stop the recidivism rate by giving these kids another way to deal with the frustration, fear, and pain they experience. To teach them that you can't always change the things you don't like, but you can always change how you let them affect you—that's where your power is.

"Racism in this country is not as overt as it once was, but it has not ended," says Krishna, whose teaching of yoga is frequently framed in the context of what it means to be black in

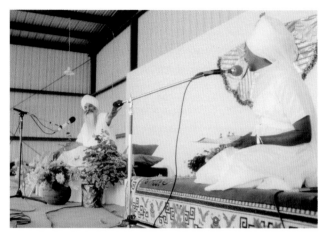

Krishna with her guru, Yogi Bhajan, at the annual Peace Prayer Day in Espanola, New Mexico, in 1989.

America. "People ask me, 'Why do you need a black yoga teachers association? Yoga's not about black and white.' Well no, it's not. But why do you have yoga retreats for just women? Because you want to focus on areas that are important to certain groups of people. No yoga association says 'white only,' but that doesn't mean black people feel included. There are no images that look like you anywhere. No one has your butt, your lips, the color of your skin. Show me a picture of yoga pos-

2. Westerners spend so much time sitting in chairs we tend to lose the full range of motion natural to the hip and knee joints. Squatting poses reclaim the health of these joints and of the complex muscles surrounding them. Place your feet mat-width apart and parallel as you lower the buttocks toward the floor and press your upper arms or elbows into your inner knees. If you cannot keep your heels down, place a folded blanket or mat beneath them and let your steady, calm breath relax you deeper into the pose ❸. And remember: As is true for most postures, if taking this shape is difficult for you, that means you need to do it.

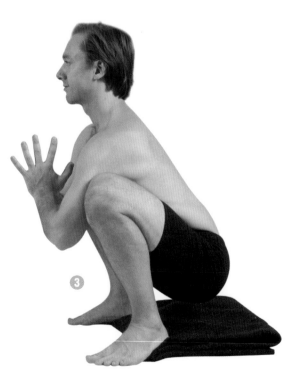

ture that doesn't have a skinny white person doing it and maybe more people of color can relate!

"When yoga was practiced in ancient days, people didn't go to a class for an hour with a gym bag and then walk down the street and get a cappuccino. It was a personal approach to: How do you do life? So we learn these tools not simply to perfect the best Headstand or chant the longest mantra or hold the greatest meditation, but to affect how we deal with what comes up in our lives."

Like many of Yogi Bhajan's early devotees, Krishna adopted not only his practice but his faith, by becoming a Sikh, or "student of truth." The five-hundred-year-old religion professes that there is more than one way to worship the divine and that they are all perfect—which suits Krishna to a T. "It doesn't really matter what style of yoga you do," she says. "Pick the style that's comfortable to you and go. These traditions are like the sticks you tie plants to when they're young, so they can survive

3. The flexibility gained through squatting is coupled with strength in Fierce pose, or *Utkatasana*, which is basic to, but done differently in, many styles of practice. The Kripalu tradition favors keeping the feet hip-width apart and the arms parallel alongside the ears ④. In Astanga Yoga, the feet and knees are together with the palms pressed into a prayer overhead ⑤. Either way, keep the pelvic floor toned, the knees over the toes, and the lower back long as you sit deeply and lift the heart.

the wind and rain until they're strong enough to hold their own shape.

"Religion is like that, too, and meditation. They both provide a certain form, a ceremonial dance that keeps you in the flow of your spiritual development. There will come a time when you will become so connected you'll no longer need the specifics of that form. And once you get to the top of the mountain, it doesn't matter what mode you have used—if you flew, took a bus, drove your car, or got out and walked. It doesn't matter. You got there."

BREATH OF FIRE

The rapid sniffing inhalation and exhalation known as Breath of Fire is standard practice in a Kundalini class. Like *Kapalabhati* (p. 186), Breath of Fire is accomplished by strong, rhythmic movement of the diaphragm. The difference is that here the inhalations and exhalations are the same length, and both are shallow and quick. The breathing technique is invigorating, purifying, and strengthening.

"When you stimulate the breath this way, you take more oxygen into the body, which forces the body to create more red blood cells to move the oxygen through," Krishna Kaur says. "That enhances circulation. The heat or 'fire' that is generated is said to eliminate toxins, some of which are excreted through perspiration. The practice can also increase the benefit and duration of poses.

"While you're holding a posture, there is always someplace where it is focusing a stress, which acts as kind of a pressure point on some system of the body—a gland, an organ, or a meridian. When we add Breath of Fire, that concentration of pressure is stimulated further. Also, in held postures, your muscles begin to throw out lactic acid, which tires them out and makes you think, Oh, this is enough! But because you're moving more oxygen through the body with such rapid motion, the toxins get flushed and you gain the ability to sustain the posture longer, providing a greater opportunity to benefit from the pressure point being activated."

Maintain a calm, steady *drishti,* or gaze, as you keep the practice going in whatever pose you are holding. *Ardha Navasana* (p. 41), *Purvottanasana* (p. 137), and its variation, Tabletop, are commonly taught with Breath of Fire. In all of these poses, relaxed concentration will allow you to build endurance.

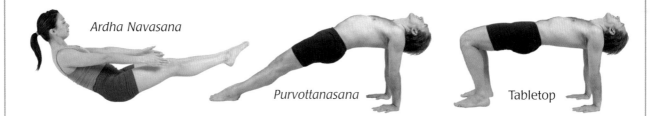

Ardha Navasana

Purvottanasana

Tabletop

"Getting into and out of the poses quickly doesn't give them a chance to stimulate what they're meant to stimulate," Krishna says. "The difference can be experienced over time. When you're starting, you may be able to hold the pose for thirty seconds. That's fine, because you get enough to begin to benefit from the pose. But once everything grows stronger, it will take longer to get the same kind of stimulation. We usually hold postures with Breath of Fire between a minute and a half and three minutes, which is a good time frame to allow these systems to be activated."

Perhaps more than with any other *pranayama* technique, the sweetest lesson from Breath of Fire comes when you release it. Be sure to practice all *pranayama* the way it has traditionally been taught, with sufficient repose afterward to allow yourself to feel what you have experienced.

4. Twisting in *Utkatasana* boosts equilibrium while opening the shoulders, chest, and spine. Keep the seat low and the hips level as you turn your torso to the left, bracing your right elbow outside your left knee or thigh 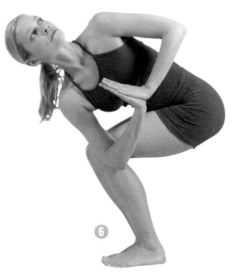. Press your palms together in front of the heart, with the left elbow pointed toward the ceiling and the right elbow aimed at the floor. Check to make sure your right knee doesn't sneak forward of your left, which indicates unevenness in the hips. Draw your shoulders back and down, and twist subtly deeper on each exhale. Repeat on the right side.

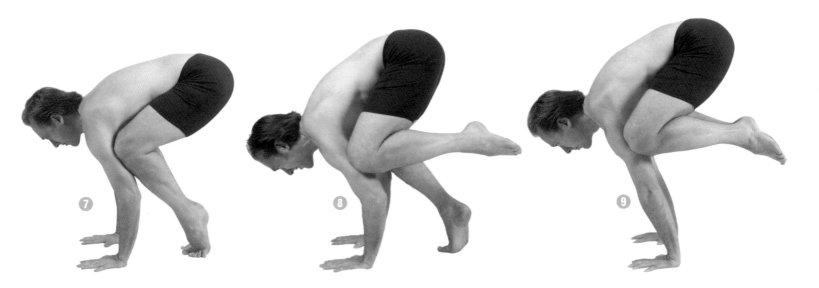

5. Bring balance into the mix by moving into Crane pose (also known as Crow), or *Bakasana*. From Frog pose lean forward and place your palms on the floor under your shoulders. Then lift your hips and place your knees on the backs of your upper arms ➐. Transfer your weight onto your hands as you squeeze your upper arms with your inner knees, and try lifting your feet off the floor one at a time ➑. To gain the lightness and strength you need to lift both feet off the floor ➒, apply *uddiyana* and *mula bandha*. Keep a steady, relaxed gaze at a point slightly in front of your hands and breathe into your back muscles.

Rodney Yee

Warrior Two
(Virabhadrasana II)

Rodney Yee wants to practice what he does not know. "When great musicians play, they're asking a question, listening for the sound, and matching it, so it's an alive philosophy," he says. "That to me is what yoga is all about."

Rodney was a physical therapy–philosophy major at the University of California at Davis when he took a ballet class after being "blown away" by a dance performance he had seen. A year later he was performing with the Oakland Ballet. "In 1977 women had to train for ballet their whole life, but if you were a man and knew which foot was left and which was right, you could practically be onstage," Rodney says. A gymnast since childhood, he had always had an athletic but tight body, which ballet exacerbated. Although it had never occurred to him to take yoga, a class was being held on the floor just above the dance studio where he studied, and he decided to see what it had to offer.

"It was one of the most amazing experiences I'd had in my life," Rodney says. "I came away thinking, It's legal to feel this way?" The class was taught by an Iyengar Yoga teacher who knew the body extremely well, "which to a dancer is important," Rodney notes. "That was an immediate turn-on. I felt more emotionally cleansed and physically balanced than I had from anything I had ever done." From then on he managed to fit yoga into what had become a full-time performance schedule. When he moved to Tokyo to dance with the Matsuyama Ballet Company in 1983, a yoga teacher who chanced to be in the company enabled Rodney to continue exploring the practice. By the time he returned to the Bay Area the following year, his dedication to ballet had given way to an interest in jazz and

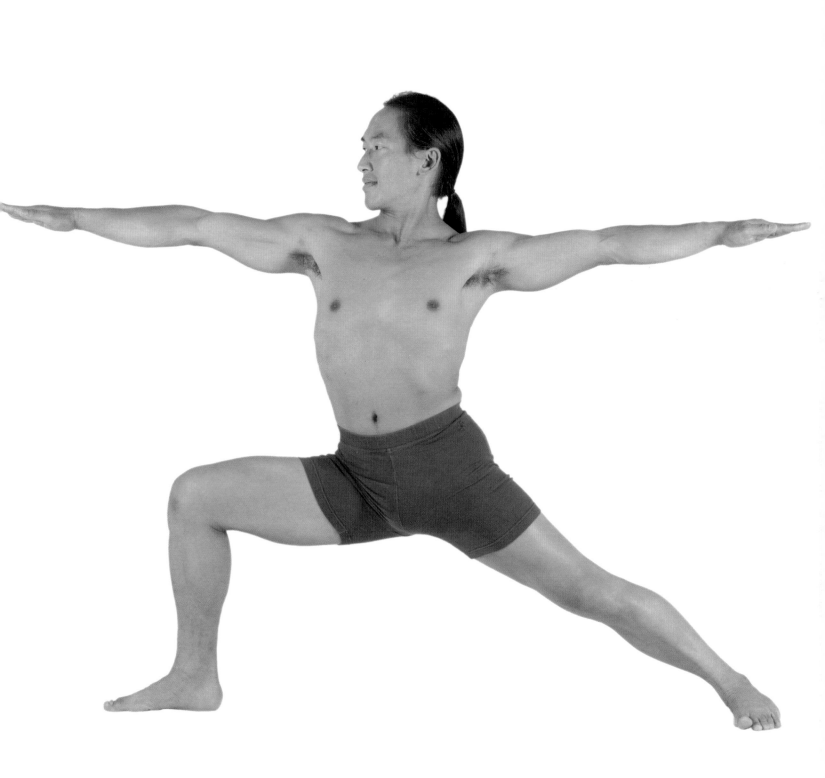

modern dance and, increasingly, to yoga. In 1985 yoga entirely supplanted his dance career.

Rodney began taking teacher-training courses at the San Francisco Iyengar Yoga Institute as a way to deepen his practice. But he was ultimately driven to share his love for the ancient discipline, and so he began to teach it, together with his wife, Donna Fone, in their apartment. "We would clear away the furniture and invite our friends over. In a year we had twenty students." In 1987 Rodney, Donna, and two other Iyengar teachers opened the Piedmont Yoga Studio in Oakland, which the couple still codirects. That same year, when B.K.S.

Iyengar was in the Bay Area conducting workshops, Rodney took his first class with the master.

"It was extraordinary," Rodney says. "I didn't know that the human body could be mapped out that deeply, that someone could understand it that well and make clear how the mind and breath are intertwined. Everybody thinks Iyengar is a physical yogi, but the beginning of meditation is concentration. If you're spreading your toes while you're dropping the groin and deepening the tailbone and keeping your collarbones open and energizing the heart *chakra* and quieting the brain and relaxing the inner ears and grounding the

THE YOGA OF THE POSE: "When there's complete organic synthesis and you're feeling everything at once, you're just this archetypal shape that's surging up from the earth. It's like every so often you see a tree that's incredibly balanced. It doesn't mean it's perfect or symmetrical, but it's just balanced, and you think, Yeah, that's a tree. You don't see one part of it—'Oh, that tree has a big branch to the right' or 'That tree is falling over'—you just see tree."

HOW STUDENTS COMMONLY MISS IT: "By becoming obsessed with doing things right instead of feeling the magnificent interchange of what's taking place in the moment—the vibration with the earth, the vibration of their feet with their arms, their legs with their spine. They're intellectualizing something, so it looks sort of right. But it has no vibrancy to it. It's a conception instead of an aliveness.

"A lot of times I see *Virabhadrasana II,* and I think, The arms are okay, the legs are okay—but where's *Virabhadrasana II*? Where's the pose? There's no synthesis. The arms are in a straight line, the front leg is at ninety degrees, the chest is lifted, the fingers are together, but you don't get the gestalt of the pose. Just like sometimes you hear music and all the parts are right, but it's not music; it's technical wizardry."

HOW TO MAKE SURE YOU CONNECT: "Get rid of your whole education, which is based on performing and on being the 'good student.' You have to be willing to feel and to fall over and to lose yourself until you become a truly good student. When you are willing to sacrifice aliveness for looking good, which most of us are, unfortunately, then that's all you get. To somebody who has a good eye, you don't even look good. You look pretend good.

"Take the chance to open the heart by listening to how you connect with the earth, then draw the energy up through your body and through the expanse of your arms. As you study the architecture and feel the flow of breath moving through the posture, continue to question the pose. Use Thich Nhat Hanh's philosophy of 'I arrive and I never arrive,' so that at the same time you feel content with what is going on now, you're constantly listening to make the pose appropriate for the ever changing moment."

femur bones—how are you not concentrating? In order to understand that much about the body, the mind has to be so beautiful in its presence; it has to be listening, feeling, experimenting, and questioning, as Iyengar's always is."

In 1987 Rodney and Donna went to Pune, India, for six weeks of public classes with Iyengar and his daughter, Geeta; they returned for a three-week training intensive in 1989. What Rodney learned there altered his approach indelibly. "Iyengar Yoga to me means to be willing to go inside your own body and do your own home-work, which becomes an incredibly creative process," he says. "Unfortunately, people use Iyengar's discoveries as the Ten Commandments instead of realizing that his real discovery was having the integrity and the courage to find out the truth for himself in this moment. He's a genius, and people are going to follow a genius. But if you're just trying to jam your body into his words, into his vibrations, you're not doing Iyengar Yoga. You're not doing yoga at all."

Propelled by his own particular genius, Rodney is able to fine-tune students' sensibilities until everyone in the room is engaged in a spiritu-al and physical ballet of exploration. By 1990 he was teaching at studios and conference work-shops in the United States as well as internation-ally. Within a few years he was one of America's best-known yoga teachers and probably its most visible one.

Eventually Rodney became less entrenched in the institution of Iyengar Yoga. "I still teach very much in the Iyengar tradition as it was taught in the '80s, which was with the understanding that people need to get in their bodies and move," he says. "In many Iyengar classes now, there's too much explanation too early on, so that people are receiving detailed information before having experiential phenomena. That is how Iyengar trains teachers, but it's not how he teaches class-es." In Rodney's studies with Manouso Manos and Ramanand Patel, two early and influential Iyengar

teachers in the Bay Area, practice was active. "We'd be swimming on our mats. Sometimes we would do one hundred and eight Sun Salutations or twenty-one standing poses twice on each side, a minute to a side. One day it was someone's forty-third birthday, so we did forty-three back-bends."

Rodney's own teaching has shifted to encom-pass "deeper relaxation with more vigorous work," he says. "It is so different from when I first began. I'm much more interested in letting the breath, mind, and body create a synthesis, and in not going so fast that you can't be aware of whether that's happening."

As his personal practice increasingly compris-es sitting meditation, he continues to examine how that ties in with asana and *pranayama*. "Posture is an extremely important part of medita-tion. To understand the intricacies and placement of your body, to make the body a house for the breath to flow easily and for the mind to be pres-ent in every cell, to be able to move on a very sub-tle, intuitive, and almost unconscious level—not unmindfully, but in the sense that your body is responding almost by itself—is so integral. Then we can begin to bring the *yamas* and *niyamas* (p. 56) into our practice and our life in a way that illu-minates and celebrates who we are. It's living in the philosophy. It's asking questions, not just thinking, Okay, nonviolence. Well, what is nonvio-lence? What is it right now—in my mind, in my body, in my actions? How does it show up? It becomes an ongoing question. The question is so deep that it keeps making you be present with yourself."

Rodney did not complete his degree in physi-cal therapy, a decision he doesn't regret. "Science looks at the body as if you can actually under-stand it, and the more I learn about the body, the more it's like a huge mystery," he says. "A podia-trist once told me, 'You can't really change the shape of your foot,' and I said, 'What are you talk-ing about?' That is what's difficult to me about

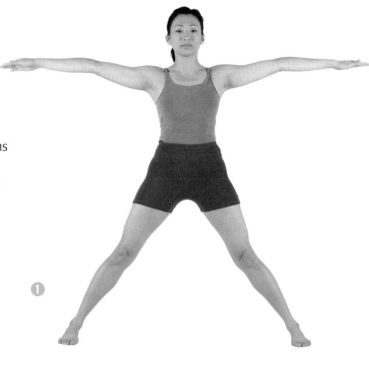

Practicing Warrior Two
(Virabhadrasana II)

1. Stand with your feet wide enough apart so that when you extend your arms, your ankles are under your forearms or wrists ❶. In this preparatory pose, which Kripalu Yoga calls Five-Pointed Star, begin to "listen to how you connect with the earth," as Rodney recommends. Turn your right foot out 90 degrees and your left foot in 45 degrees ❷, then use the strength of your outer left leg to bend your right knee over your right ankle ❸. Keep attempting to bring your front femur bone parallel to the floor while remaining aware of its relationship to the groundedness of the back leg.

being a teacher: Experience can sometimes cloud your vision. That's exactly why people like Iyengar and Einstein are so brilliant. Because as much experience and brilliance as they have, they see new again and again, like little kids. They keep coming back to the beginner's mind."

For all his admiration of the man he calls "the Einstein of yoga," Rodney never considered Iyengar his guru in the traditional sense of the word. "Some people need to follow a guru, and the *Bhagavad Gita* says that kind of devotion is one of the paths to enlightenment. But while I'm devoted to the practice, I haven't found a person so overwhelmingly connected to God that I feel I need to drop into them in order to find that connection. Tomorrow I might be saying something totally different, but right now this is where I land.

For people who feel totally devoted to their guru—it's one of the most beautiful things I've seen in my life."

Rodney continues to listen deeply to the guru within and to find it everywhere without. "As my understanding of yoga increases—as it has, I hope, over twenty-three years—I want to share it," he says. "What makes a great yoga teacher is to have a wealth of knowledge, yet be willing to just completely let that go and in some sense ad-lib—without all the trappings of your own life. I'm more interested than ever in looking at what's here and what's there, in taking other people's classes. I am more confused and more full of questions in some ways than ever. And I'm happy to be happy in that state."

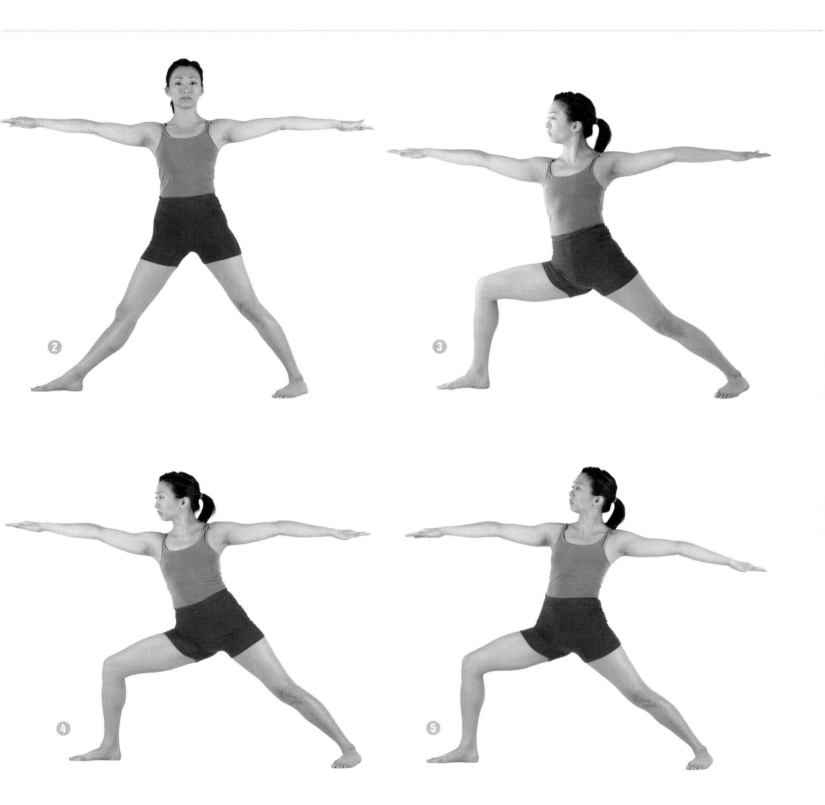

2. "Students in America tend to lean in the direction they're going, moving into the future all the time," Rodney notes. "Others lean toward the back arm and leg, which represent the past." So bring yourself into the center by intentionally moving out of it. Shift your torso alternately right ❹ and left ❺. Then bring your shoulders directly over your hips and sit deeply into the pose ❸ as you draw energy up through your spine, which Rodney says aligns you with the present moment.

Warrior Two *(Virabhadrasana II)*

3. From Warrior Two slide your left hand down your outer left thigh and reach your right arm over your ear for an intense side opening ⓺ that is also a lovely preparation for Extended Side Angle *(Utthita Parsvakonasana)* ⓻.
In the fullest expression of *Parsvakonasana,* the Warrior Two foundation stays firm and true as you press your right palm on the floor outside your right foot and shoot your left arm over your ear. But if your torso faces the floor instead of the wall in front of you, you need to work with a block inside ⓼ or outside your foot so you keep length in both sides of your body. With or without a block, keep lifted through the arch of the left foot and grounded through its outer edge, and spin your ribs toward the ceiling. Resist your right shoulder with your right knee to keep the right thighbone emerging straight out of its socket and parallel to the floor.

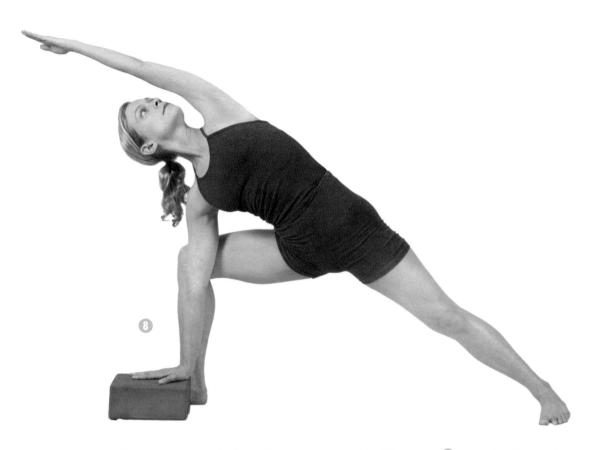

4. If you are comfortable in *Parsvakonasana,* bind the pose ⑨ into what the Viniyoga tradition calls a fixed-frame twist, "in which the arms are used as levers to maximize the rotation of the spine and shoulders," as Gary Kraftsow explains. Thread your left arm under your thigh and reach your right arm behind your back, catching the top wrist with the bottom hand. Remember that the purpose of binding is its concomitant expansion; if all you feel is restriction, let it go and return to the variation where you experienced a sense of spaciousness.

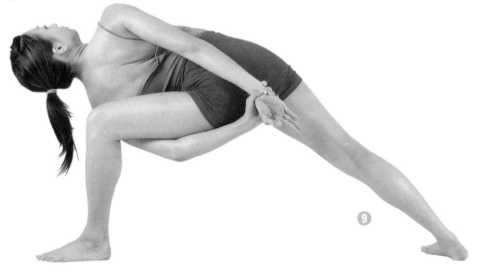

Judith Hanson Lasater
Extended Triangle
(Utthita Trikonasana)

Judith Hanson Lasater wants everybody to relax. For more than three decades she has investigated, taught, discussed, and written about yoga asanas, but what interests her now is aligning students with each pose's true purpose—to remind us that we are already whole. "The philosophical underpinning of yoga is that you are complete in and of yourself," she says. "When you understand that, when there's nowhere to go and nothing to do, you can approach asanas with deep self-respect, non-competition, and a sense of fun and exploration."

Judith came to yoga in 1970 as a twenty-three-year-old graduate student with an increasingly debilitating case of arthritis. After her first class, at the Austin, Texas, YMCA, she sensed that asana practice would prove as important to her spiritually as physically. "Not only did I instantly feel better, but I came away with the realization that these poses are forms of worship," she says. She has not been bothered by arthritis since, a miracle she attributes to heightened immune system function brought about by yoga, a change in diet that included fasting, and falling in love with her future husband—not necessarily in that order.

Ten months after Judith's first class, the instructor at the Austin Y left, and with no training whatsoever Judith Hanson the yoga student became Judith Hanson the yoga teacher. Judith was not concerned, since she had taken class for the better part of a year and figured she knew everything there was to know. Then she sat down in front of her first class and froze, as she recalls. "What was I going to say? What was I going to do? Oh, my God, what had I gotten myself into? So I took a deep breath and suddenly had this incredible

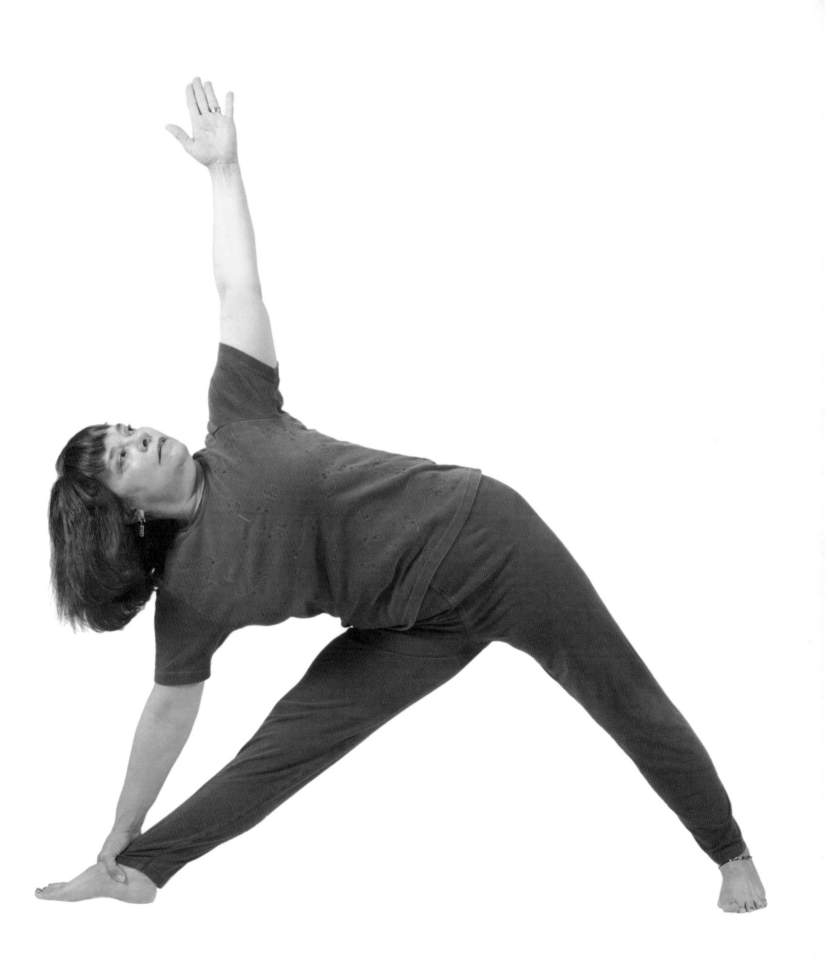

Extended Triangle *(Utthita Trikonasana)*

THE YOGA OF THE POSE: "The triangle, or pyramid, is a powerful and ancient archetype. Pyramids are thousands and thousands of years old, yet they stand against all kinds of things because of their deep stability. They connect us to the earth and point us toward heaven. So in *Trikonasana,* from the center of my belly I feel the feminine, or *shakti,* energy going down, which to me is experiencing God as imminent right here and now. Then I have my arms and heart lifting for the heavens in a longing to connect with deity as a transcendent.

"On a physical basis *Trikonasana* encourages and maintains healthy function of the legs and hips, which is important for people in our culture who sit a lot. It facilitates free movement of the pelvis in walking and standing and lifting. It stretches out the back. It opens the chest. The arms make a very exuberant, thrown-open-wide kind of movement I like very much. I'm wide, I'm planted, I'm stable, there's a slight backbend; and it requires a certain amount of balance. So it's almost a mini yoga session."

HOW STUDENTS COMMONLY MISS IT:
"By taking it too seriously—thinking, If I get *Trikonasana* just right, then my life will be just right. Or by not taking it seriously enough, because if you don't practice *Trikonasana* with love and attention, you cannot reap its benefits.

"Many students think *Trikonasana* is when they've gone down into the pose. They don't understand that the pose is the intention and the movement as you go into it and the clarity and awareness as you come out, as much as it is being 'in it.' So they miss it that way. They think that there's something to achieve instead of something to enjoy.

"People tend not to allow enough freedom in the back hip. They're focused on the front hip because that's what's in front, what they see, where they're going, where the future is, what's next. But the back leg and hip represent our stability, our launching pad, the intention from which we create the action. When we are equally present with the action of the back hip, we are more likely to be present as we move forward. Yet the way most practitioners open the back hip is by holding back the pelvis and the thigh together, which actually shuts it down."

HOW TO MAKE SURE YOU CONNECT: "Give up the idea of 'getting it' and stay focused on being present with the experience of it. In other words, be present with the numbers you're adding up. If you're going for the sum, you probably won't get the answer. You'll make a mistake because you won't be focused on what you're doing.

"In the beginning emphasize three things: Bring your front knee out so that the kneecap points over the little toe. Keep your legs completely straight. And breathe—as you move in, as you stay, and as you come out. If you don't feel stable, stand with your feet a little closer together or do the pose against the wall. Allow your back hip to open by externally rotating your back leg and knee, and letting the rim of the pelvis move slightly forward. This accommodates the natural arch in the lumbar spine. The most beautiful poses are those that reflect the natural laws of movement and the natural lines of the body.

"So move into and out of the pose with gently directed awareness. The asana is not an answer; it's a question. If you approach *Trikonasana* as an exploration, as a possibility instead of a goal to be achieved, there's no way to miss anything."

image of my teacher standing right behind me and her teacher behind her, all the way back into an infinity of teachers standing one behind the other. I realized I was just the water carrier, bringing the next bucket of water to put out the fire. It wasn't me at all. It didn't matter what I said as long as I let the water flow."

Judith began to perceive the force of that flow—and of her neophyte status in conducting it—when she took a workshop with Bernard Rishi and Karen Stephen, two senior students of the yoga master B.K.S. Iyengar. "I immediately loved the system," she says. "It was precise and clear and had such internal integrity." Wanting to learn more about what she was teaching, Judith attended a training program led by Swami Vishnu-devananda at the Sivananda Ashram in the Bahamas—as part of her honeymoon, in January 1972. (Happily, the man she married was and is a fellow practitioner.)

"It was fascinating to study with an Indian teacher," Judith recalls. "Swami Vishnu was dedicated and energetic, and he had yoga in his blood. He'd lived in an ashram, and he was running an ashram. We learned about everything— asana, chanting, philosophy. It was a great introduction to the whole of yoga."

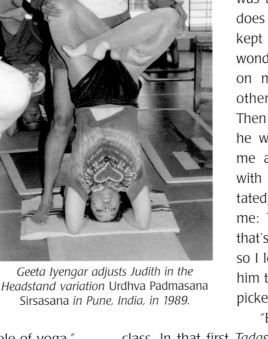

Geeta Iyengar adjusts Judith in the Headstand variation Urdhva Padmasana Sirsasana *in Pune, India, in 1989.*

Still, Judith wanted more. Her yen for learning, combined with a need for a "legitimate" profession led her to pursue training as a physical therapist. In August 1972 she and her husband packed up and moved to the San Francisco Bay area, where she immediately began teaching yoga while establishing the residency that would allow her to attend the University of California at San Francisco. Judith got involved with other yoga teachers in the area and in 1974 cofounded the California Yoga Teachers Association (CYTA), which she still heads. Together with that group she established the yoga center that was to become the San Francisco Iyengar Institute.

When Mr. Iyengar, the honorific by which his Western students religiously refer to him, came to San Francisco in the spring of 1974, Judith made sure she was up front and center on the day the workshop began. "The very first pose he taught was *Tadasana,*" she says, "and he kept verbally picking on me, saying I wasn't really doing it and why did I call myself a yoga teacher? My first reaction was to get a little angry: Who does this guy think he is? He kept doing it, and I started wondering, Why is he picking on me? There are thirty-five other people in this room! Then all of a sudden I got it— he was using asana to teach me about the way I interact with the world. First I get irritated, then I go to poor-little-me: Those are my strategies; that's my inner dialogue. And so I looked at him and flashed him this big grin, and he never picked on me again.

"But I'll never forget the class. In that first *Tadasana* he would say things like, 'Your feet are *bhakti* yogis [yogis of devotion] that caress the earth. Your thighs are karma yogis [yogis of action] that do the work of holding up the body. He went through all these different yogas in the body in that one pose. I thought, Here is someone who really gets it. And I was sold." By fall she and several other attendees were teaching Iyengar-style yoga.

Extended Triangle *(Utthita Trikonasana)*

As yoga and spirituality took center stage in Judith's work, she chose not to enter into practice as a physical therapist. In 1975 she and five other CYTA members launched *Yoga Journal.* In addition to her regular column for the magazine, she had a heavy teaching schedule, received her Ph.D. in East-West psychology, and made three sojourns to Iyengar's school in Pune, India. And she gave birth to three children.

Judith took her last trip to Pune in 1989. "I'm in another stage," she says, "and that's not about rejecting my teachers but more about saying yes to myself. Technique is necessary—if you want to play the piano, you have to learn how to read music and press the keys—but you can know everything there is to know about *Trikonasana* and

still be miserable. My study now is what the pose can teach me about living fully in this moment, and about how I integrate life into yoga and yoga into life."

Does she practice and teach asanas the Iyengar way? "It's really hard to say, because I feel that the process is an evolution," Judith notes. "To insist a pose is absolutely done one way—Mr. Iyengar himself doesn't do that. He's always changing. So in some ways there isn't an Iyengar method, there's just B.K.S. Iyengar doing yoga. We're the ones who aren't convinced we know something unless it's set in concrete. To study yoga is to be willing to let go of your safety so you—and others—can challenge your beliefs about how you think life is. Because that's when you

Practicing Extended Triangle *(Utthita Trikonasana)*

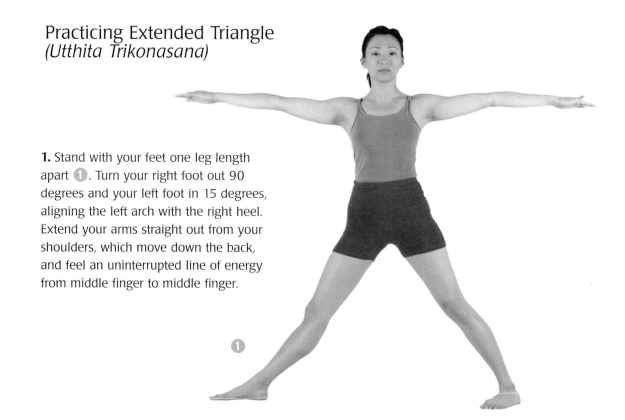

1. Stand with your feet one leg length apart ❶. Turn your right foot out 90 degrees and your left foot in 15 degrees, aligning the left arch with the right heel. Extend your arms straight out from your shoulders, which move down the back, and feel an uninterrupted line of energy from middle finger to middle finger.

grow, when you're a little bit challenged. When I use the asana to challenge my beliefs of who I think I am physically, mentally, emotionally, I open up to a new way of being in the world." And that, the veteran teacher explains, should include being open to a new way of practice.

"There may be a time when two hours a day of asana is not enough and other times when thirty minutes is enough," Judith says. "There may be a time we require an all-restorative practice or a lot of meditation. The question is what do I need right now in order to be present? And then not just to be present—that's the beginning of spiritual life—but to become radically present and alive to this moment, so I can then choose actions that create the results I want in the world and create the world I want to live in and leave behind.

"We Americans have lost the gentleness, consistency, and direction of the practice. And what has taken its place is ambition. When I started practicing yoga, there weren't that many people doing it, but they were really committed. Now it's about a mile wide and an inch deep. Everyone thinks they know what yoga is, but I believe many of us have conflated asana with yoga. Yoga is about deep Self-inquiry into the nature of the mind. *Svadhyaya,* or Self-study, asana, *pranayama,* meditation, taking *darshana* with a guru—these are the ways to open our heart and to become free of the dominance of judgment and thought. And that's the practice. Standing on my head is important because of the residue of

2. Draw the right hip back as you reach out toward the right on an inhale ②; then move the right arm down and the left arm up as you exhale and take the shape of Triangle ③. Different styles of practice dictate alternate placement of the bottom hand and a different distance between the feet. Be willing to try a new way, Judith advises. "See what happens," she says. "See where you're limited, see where you're free—with the idea that as soon as you're convinced you know, you're lost."

②   ③

Extended Triangle *(Utthita Trikonasana)*

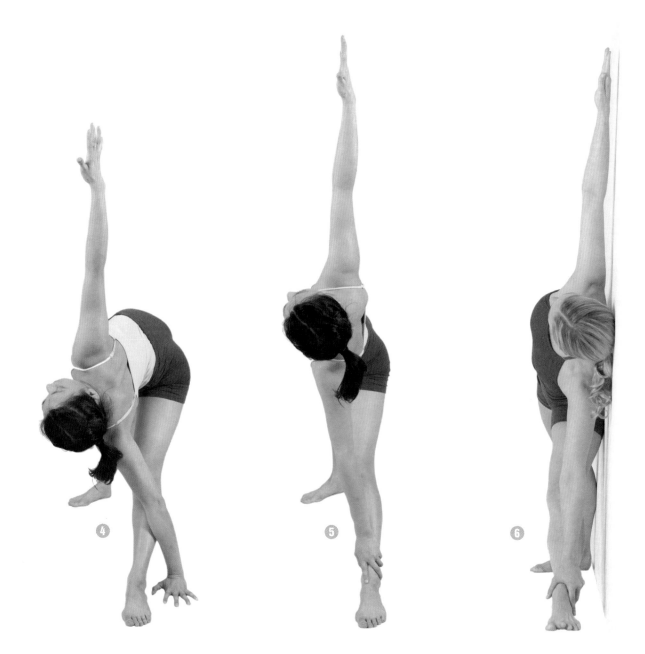

3. The palm-on-the-floor variation shown in ❸, often associated with the Iyengar tradition, is fine if you have flexible hamstrings and hips. But if it causes your ribs to hang forward of your thigh and your buttocks to stick out behind you ❹, you have moved away from the intelligence of the pose and into the sort of misperception we are practicing to avoid. So raise your hand up to your ankle or shin until you feel an expanse of energy from shoulder to shoulder and from your tailbone to the crown of your head ❺. Working against the wall ❻ is a good way to gain understanding of this alignment, and it also offers support for older practitioners or those who have trouble balancing.

4. The Astanga Yoga *Trikonasana* ⑦ classically involves a shorter stance that allows you to catch your right big toe in yogic toe lock (p. 26). But Richard Freeman advises holding the toe only if you can do so without shutting the pose down by collapsing into it (see ④). Otherwise, he says, holding the foot, ankle, or shin will do nicely.

5. Triangle is all about length in the Sivananda tradition ⑧, which generally teaches it as the last pose to be done before final relaxation, or *Savasana.* Reach your left arm over your ear and breathe space into the intercostal muscles between the ribs.

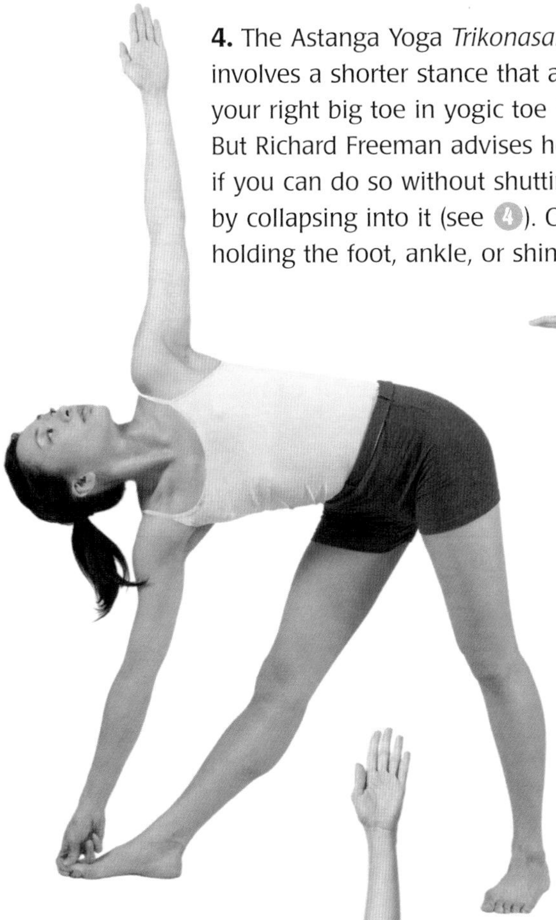

⑦

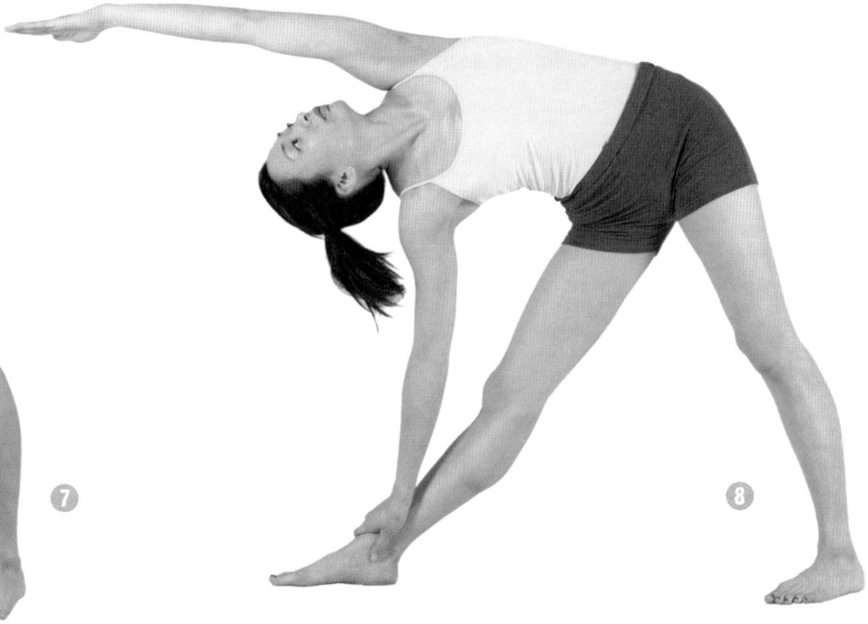

⑧

6. For the Bikram Triangle ⑨, the feet are at least four feet apart in a heel-to-heel intersection, with the right foot turned out 90 degrees and the left foot pointed straight ahead. Bend your right knee over your ankle and bring the femur bone parallel to the floor. Tilt the torso until your right elbow presses against your right knee and the fingertips graze the floor in front of your toes, creating a triangle between your right arm, thigh, and ribcage. Move your left hip down and forward as you take your left arm, ribs, and shoulder up and back. Raise your chin toward your left shoulder and look up.

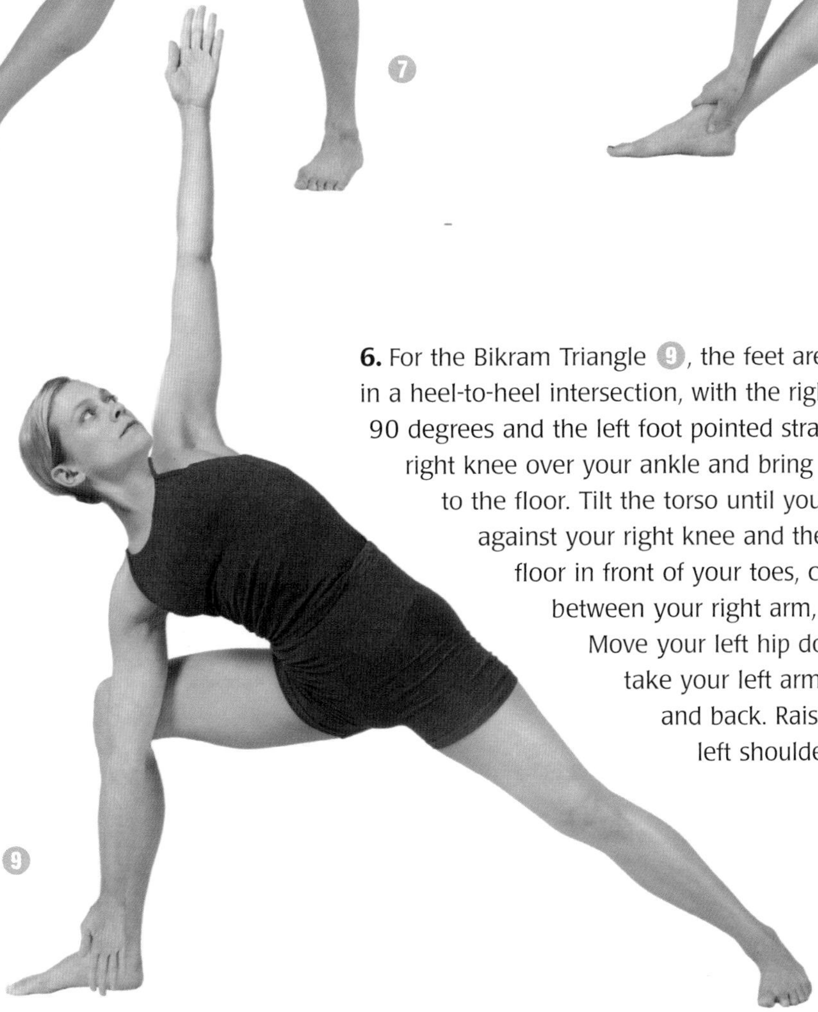

⑨

awareness it leaves in my body and soul; but really, who cares if I can stand on my head—can I live my life with an open heart? If my asana practice is not fulfilling that, if it's not encouraging the river of being present to grow and flow in my life, then it's not working."

What works for Judith today is to cull the essence of Corpse pose, or *Savasana,* and bring it into whatever practice she is teaching or doing. It's a lesson America is evidently hungry to receive,

judging from the waiting lists that accrue at yoga centers nationwide for her workshops in restorative yoga. "As you relax the body," Judith says, "you observe the breath, you observe your thoughts, and you begin to see that you are not your thoughts. Instead of saying, 'I am angry,' you say, 'I am having an angry thought,' which is hugely different. There's a tenth of an inch between heaven and hell, and that's the tenth of an inch—and it is the beginning of freedom."

7. To move into Revolved Triangle *(Parivrtta Trikonansa)* ⑩, step your right foot back two and a half to three feet, and angle the back foot nearly parallel to the front foot. Go for a heel-to-heel intersection to start. Square your hips toward your front leg, take your left hand to your left hip, and inhale your right arm up alongside your ear.

8. As you exhale, draw the left hip back and bow forward until your torso and right arm are parallel to the floor ⑪. Move your shoulders toward your hips as you extend your right fingertips toward the wall in front of you. This is a fine place to work if the next step is not yet possible for you.

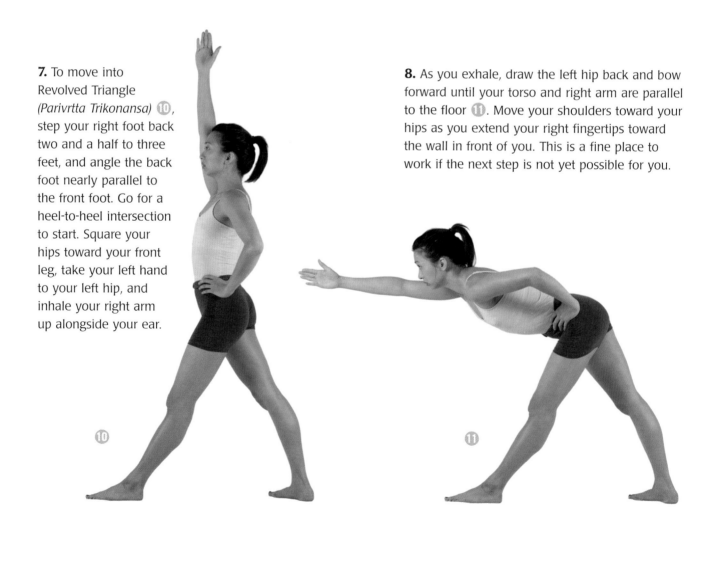

9. Place your right hand on the floor outside your left foot and lift your left arm up to the ceiling, stacking the shoulders and wrists one on top of the other ⑫. A common instruction is to keep both hips square to the floor and initiate the twist at the waist. But Judith encourages students to drop the right hip slightly to allow the pelvis to move with the twist—to avoid injuries that twists like this (see p. 118) can engender or exacerbate.

10. In order to be stable enough to open into the twisting balance of *Parivrtta Trikonansa*, you must be grounded through your left foot, your right hand, and the outer edge of your right foot. So if you cannot root the palm of your right hand into the floor, use a block ⑬ or even the back of a chair to gain the benefits of the pose.

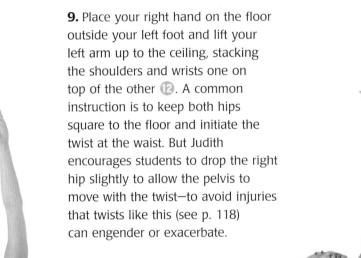

John Friend

Half Moon
(Ardha Chandrasana)

John Friend's first yoga teacher was a woman who never practiced an asana in her life: his mother. When he was a young boy, she tried to satisfy his curiosity about the mysteries of existence. "When I was eight, she read me stories about yogis from *Fate* magazine" (a publication whose own stated mission, then as now, is "honest reporting and open discussion of the strange and unknown") "and to me they were superheroes, better than the comics," John says. Seeing his keen interest, she went on to buy him his first hatha yoga books.

In the blue-collar town of Youngstown, Ohio, where John grew up, such spiritual interests made him a bit of an odd fellow at school. But when he was twelve, an older boy who had a black belt in martial arts showed him "dramatic demonstrations with a bathroom scale," whereby, using *prana,* or *qi,* as he called it, he could increase and decrease his weight by five pounds at will. "I thought, This is incredible!" John recalls. "He possessed a power that went way beyond muscle."

Within the year John was exploring those forces himself by practicing asanas from books by Swami Satchidananda, Indra Devi, Richard Hittleman, and Lilias Folan, whom he also watched on TV. At sixteen, having discovered the writings of Madame Blavatsky and Annie Besant on the shelves of his mother's library, John joined the local branch of the Theosophical Society, where he served as librarian and took his first asana classes.

John went on to study physics at the University of Cincinnati and finance and accounting at Texas A&M, where he matriculated in 1979. One day in 1980 the teacher at the

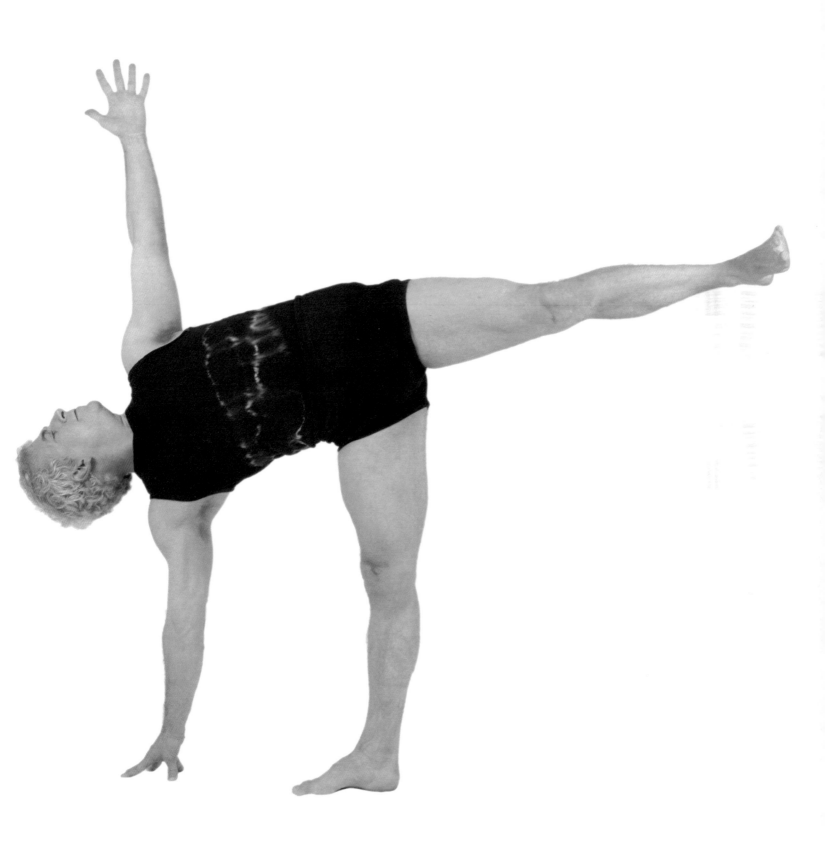

Half Moon *(Ardha Chandrasana)*

THE YOGA OF THE POSE: "Your arms are open, your legs are open, your heart is open, and you're balancing on one leg and one hand. So it's this fine line between extremely stable power to the core—where there's recognition and remembrance of your greatness, your divine nature—and then a shining out of that. The name of the pose, like the pose itself, is radiant, a balance between half light and half dark, between recognition of the individual and the reflection of the universal.

"Even someone new to yoga looks at it and they're inspired; their heart really opens by seeing someone just playing the edge in this balancing pose and then looking up at the sky. It's a great form of spiritual art."

HOW STUDENTS COMMONLY MISS IT: "There is a goodness, a beauty, an intelligence that's already there in the pose, but students can inhibit it in a couple of ways. One, they don't fully engage their muscles, in particular the muscles of the supporting leg. Maybe they're afraid of falling over—which is understandable—and in that fear they kind of disengage. They don't play the edge fully, which you have to do. This is not a casual practice. It takes an intensity to open up the middle, to focus the fullness of attention one way and the fullness of openness the other way.

"The pose starts from the foundation, that part of the body that touches the floor. What some students do is lose what they have established when they turn their head and attention upward. Another mistake people make is to try to pry the top hip open. The hip does not get pulled back; the back and the front of the top hip and the whole top leg actually get lifted straight up from an expansion that initiates at the core. That's what creates the space that allows the whole body to come into the side plane. But if you roll the top hip back, you'll jam the lower back because it's a one-sided action. And if you disengage the top leg and let the foot be lax, you lose power and current through the whole body so that you cannot be totally engaged, open, and free."

HOW TO MAKE SURE YOU CONNECT: "Do the pose in the highest sense—as a celebration of life and of yourself. Even if you fall over, which is inevitable in the course of practice, you can just laugh. You have fun. And then you get up and do it again. Every time you come back, you get stronger and stronger with the recognition that you are great, which builds on itself. So you can't fail; you can't 'do it wrong' if you smile with your eyes, with your whole inner body.

"Cultivate the pose from the ground up. Draw energy from the sole of your foot through the muscles of the supporting leg to the top of the knee by hugging and honoring your own power. Then continue the flow from the foundation into the core of the pelvis and up into the hip. The buttocks have to be engaged and the tailbone drawn deep into the body, in that same remembrance that this universal, supreme power flows through you, in your own individual form. When you understand that, it's like a self-embrace and you can suddenly hold the pose. You open the back of the body as much as the front, the underside of the body as much as the top; that's what creates the stacking of the hips. That's what allows you to open to the sun side of your Half Moon."

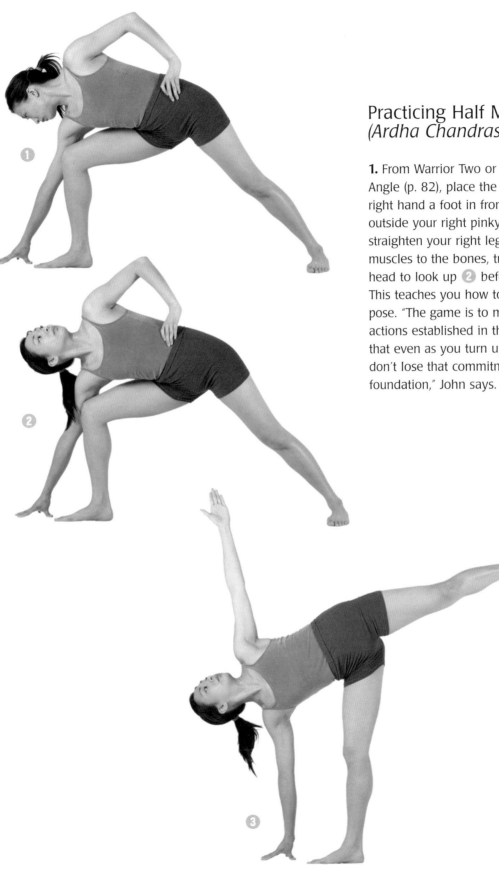

Practicing Half Moon
(Ardha Chandrasana)

1. From Warrior Two or Extended Side Angle (p. 82), place the fingertips of your right hand a foot in front of and just outside your right pinky toe ❶. As you straighten your right leg by hugging the muscles to the bones, try turning your head to look up ❷ before you lift up ❸. This teaches you how to be free in the pose. "The game is to maintain the actions established in the beginning, so that even as you turn up and go out you don't lose that commitment to your foundation," John says.

Half Moon (Ardha Chandrasana)

Houston meditation center where he had been taking an asana class got sick and asked John to teach for him. He confidently agreed. "I'd been practicing for seven years and thought I was very proficient," he says. "But when I taught my first class, I noticed everyone was doing a different pose. I realized I might have been able to do the postures, but I didn't know how to explain them. And if a student said that they had a hip problem or that something was bothering them, I just said, *'Don't move!'*" At the end of class John stood despondently at the door saying good-bye and

apologizing. But the students told him he had really maintained the spirit of yoga, which didn't make him feel all that much better, "but it made me understand that people are looking for more than just the technical aspects."

John began working as a business consultant, and continued to take and teach classes. Another Houston-area yoga teacher had studied with Doug and David Swenson, two early practitioners of K. Pattabhi Jois's Astanga Yoga, so John spent some time learning the first and second series. "It was super physically challenging," he says. "I just

2. Warrior Three ❹ is a good way to begin to explore the balance necessary for all single-leg standing postures. It is also another nice entry point for Half Moon. As you tip forward into the balance, roll your left hip down until it feels level with the right hip. Shoot energy through the back leg by flexing the foot strongly. At the same time reach through your fingertips and find a backbend feeling in the pose. To move into Half Moon, lower your right fingertips to the floor under your right shoulder and open the front of the body by pulling the left hip and leg up as you roll both your thighs in and back ❺, as John advises.

thought, This is the hardest thing you could do." Then he did something quite a bit harder.

In 1986, smack in the middle of a consulting job back in Ohio, John realized that the corporate world was not and could never be ultimately fulfilling. So he packed up his car and started driving west. "I stopped in front of a church in Indiana, got out and sat under a big oak tree," he recalls, "and I recognized that I didn't know where I was going, that nobody had any idea where I was—including me—and that I had never been that free in my entire life." He traveled around for another six months and finally headed back to Texas, where he became a full-time yoga teacher.

In his travels he had studied with Judith Lasater, whom he cites as a major influence. "I went to her advanced teachers' class—because I thought I was advanced—and she showed me how much I had to learn. The whole Iyengar system, which is what she was teaching then, was so sophisticated, I felt like I was practicing for the first time." His involvement with that discipline deepened, and in 1989 he joined a group led by Mary Dunn and journeyed to Pune, India, for a three-

3. The Bikram-style Standing Head-to-Knee builds enormous strength and stability for single-leg balancing poses by "directing energy to the specific muscles working at that moment," Emmy Cleaves (p. 120) says. Pull your right knee into your chest at waist level and interlace your fingers under your right foot ❻; then slowly and carefully begin straightening your right leg ❼, keeping your left leg straight and strong. "If you have a bad back and can't grab the foot, hold your knee and work there," Emmy Cleaves says. As you extend your top leg fully and round your head to your knee ❽, "be careful with the ligaments behind both knees," Emmy warns. "Engage the thigh muscles and keep the weight forward toward your left big toe. Check your kneecap; is it pulled up? There's a difference between just pushing the knee back so it's bone on bone and creating support with the soft tissue surrounding the knee. That's what creates strong and enduring knees."

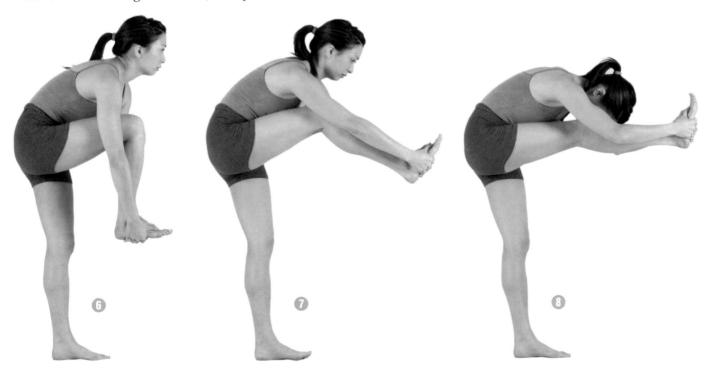

❻   ❼   ❽

week intensive with B.K.S. and Geeta Iyengar. Their instruction filled his mind with new information, but it was on a subsequent leg of his journey that he met the teacher who ignited his heart.

After touring the country awhile, John headed to the Gurudev Siddha Peeth Ashram in Ganeshpuri, established in the 1950s by the great yogi Swami Muktananda. John went to see Gurumayi Chidvilasananda, the current master of the Siddha Yoga lineage. When he approached the guru, he blurted out, "I'm from Texas, and I'm an advanced yoga practitioner, and I'd like to do a demonstration for you." She said that first thing in the morning would be fine. After ruing his hubris all night, John got up on a platform and performed a sequence of asanas that led to his teaching Gurumayi's yoga teachers—beginning the very next day.

His connection with Gurumayi was profound. "I experienced the gift of grace, or *shaktipat*, in a very tangible way," he says. "She was the strongest, most spiritually energetic and inspiring person I had ever met. And her overriding philosophy that the body, like the mind, is a manifestation of Supreme Consciousness caused a profound shift in how I was practicing yoga."

4. In Eagle pose, or *Garudasana*, we come to rest in the equilibrium between stability and freedom that John calls the key to all balancing postures. "If you grip too much, you'll get rigid and fall down, and if you're too soft and open, you'll fall down. You have to have steadfast commitment to the core or midline of the pose and at the same time allow the outside to be flexible." Step your right foot out to the right and bend both knees to set the foundation of the pose ❾ Then wrap your right leg over and around your left leg—hook your right foot around your left ankle if you can—and your right arm under and around your left arm, nestling elbow into elbow and palm into palm ❿. From here, lift your elbows until they are in line with your mouth ⓫, then bow forward and gaze out over your palms, like an eagle looking down from his aerie ⓬.

Asana had always been part of the schedule at Muktananda's ashrams—both in India and at the Shree Muktananda Ashram in South Fallsburg, New York, which the meditation master established in the late 1970s—but it was not highly emphasized until the mid-'80s. When Gurumayi took over after Muktananda's death in 1982, the hatha yoga program started to grow. With John's input and his strong Iyengar influence, Siddha yogis' attention to the details of asana increased. But it was Gurumayi who radically refined John's alignment.

"Back then I was almost attacking my practice, really trying to subjugate

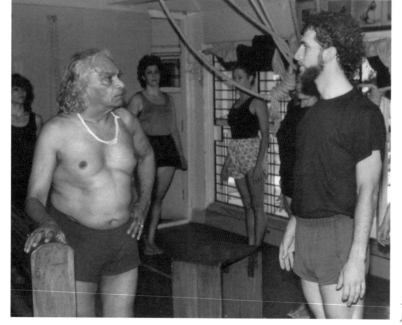

John in Pune, India, in 1989, on his first visit to study with B.K.S. Iyengar.

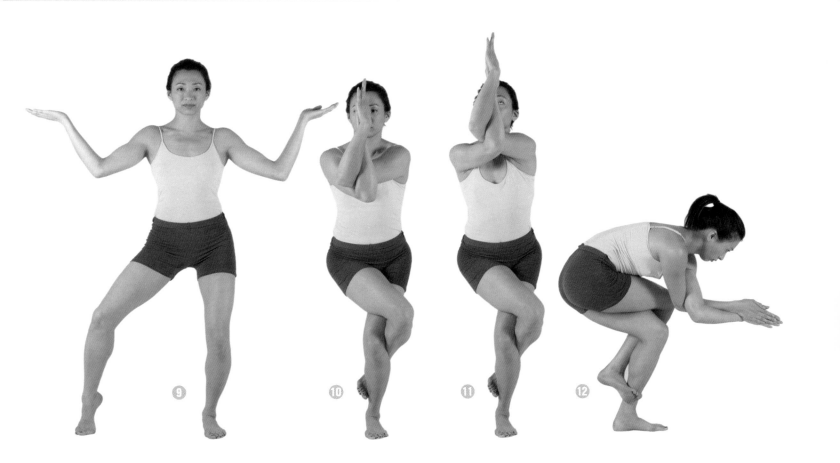

my body," John says. "She impressed on me that it's not something you're trying to dominate, but that you're trying to align yourself with this bigger flow of *shakti.* So while I was looking at imperfections to fix in my poses, her whole thing was to see the beauty. She was saying, 'There's nothing wrong with your poses. You can do them more skillfully in order to bring out more greatness.' It was so much more of an openhearted approach."

In ashram life everyone performs *seva* or selfless service. John's job was to work with teachers in the yoga department, and this job traveled with him when he went to South Fallsburg in 1991. Although John never took up permanent residence at the ashram, he performed weeks and sometimes months of service there each year and continues to do so. All the while, Iyengar Yoga remained key in what he offered at the Shree Muktananda Ashram and at his classes in The Woodlands, Texas, and in

Houston, until he returned to Pune for another Iyengar intensive in 1995.

"While I was there, I had a strong awakening that I wasn't as lined up with the Iyengar message as I was with the Siddha Yoga message," John says. He remains grateful for the knowledge he gleaned from the Iyengars, from whom he says he learned as much about *vinyasa*—the progressive connection of asanas—as he did from workshops with Pattabhi Jois, with whom that aspect of the practice is more widely associated. But the awareness that Siddha Yoga meditation deepened in him lent a whole new dimension to that facet as well.

"The idea in *vinyasa* is that you don't forget what you're doing, so it's a practice of concentration. You have to remember your divinity the whole time. When you make that your intention, the action is exactly the same throughout; there is no forgetfulness." Gurumayi exemplifies that, he says. "Her face, her gestures, the way she walks, her speaking—just picking up a glass from the table—is *vinyasa*, because she links her mind and self to every movement."

By 1997 it was clear to John, whose teaching was still associated with the Iyengar style, that he needed to indicate his change of direction. "It was a clean, natural evolution," he says. "The good things I offer definitely came from the Iyengars and all the good teachers I've had along the way. But because I had assimilated the various teachings and reinterpreted them under a whole different philosophy, it was disrespectful to call it Iyengar Yoga when it no longer was."

He notified Gurumayi of his intention to launch what he came to call Anusara Yoga, a name recommended by Douglas Brooks, a professor of religion at the University of Rochester and a visiting scholar at the ashram in Fallsburg. Anusara, from a verse in the Kashmiri scripture the *Kularnava Tantra* means to flow with grace—which has been John's guiding principle since he met Gurumayi. "When I heard the word, I thought, That's a great word for the style of hatha yoga I do," John says. "Because for me it is all about being attuned with the Supreme in every individual form, every different asana, in my breathing practice—all these things can reflect the highest within myself and the universe." Anusara Yoga

5. Side-Inclined Plane *(Vasisthasana)* recreates the openness of Half Moon while building the lateral hamstring strength that is critical to but inadequately addressed in most standing poses. From Plank pose ⑬ shift your weight onto your right palm and the outer edge of your right foot, then extend your left arm to the ceiling ⑭. Be sure you can see your left thumb with your right eye, and stack your feet. To move to a fuller expression of the posture, bend your left knee, catch the toe in yogic toe lock, and raise the left leg straight up and out ⑮.

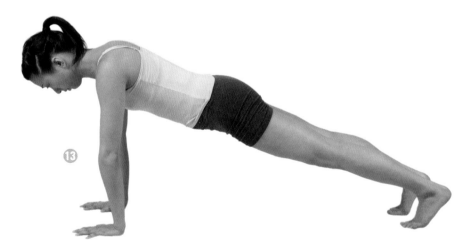

seeks to anatomically and energetically systematize that attunement, and does so with great success. There are now roughly nine hundred Anusara teachers worldwide.

This sort of branding may seem completely American—but in some ways it is as old as yoga. To John it's all as it should be. "The way I look at it is that in life and art, the creative ability to come up with diverse forms, is never-ending," John says. "So similarly, with the hatha yoga styles in the West, we can take this ancient practice and bring it into twenty-first-century Western culture in a way that can help and support everybody, really, throughout the world. It's just making it very accessible and continuing to raise the art to deeper, more sophisticated levels. That's one thing we in the West are really good at."

The teachings John has received from Gurumayi reverberate with the same message Muktananda brought to the West in the 1970s: "Respect your own Self, for God lives within you as you." It is the same message John had learned from his mother. "Honoring the best within yourself and everyone you see—that was my mom's central life philosophy," John says. And it remains the bedrock of his teachings. "Look for the good, you guys," John tells his students. "That's my big message."

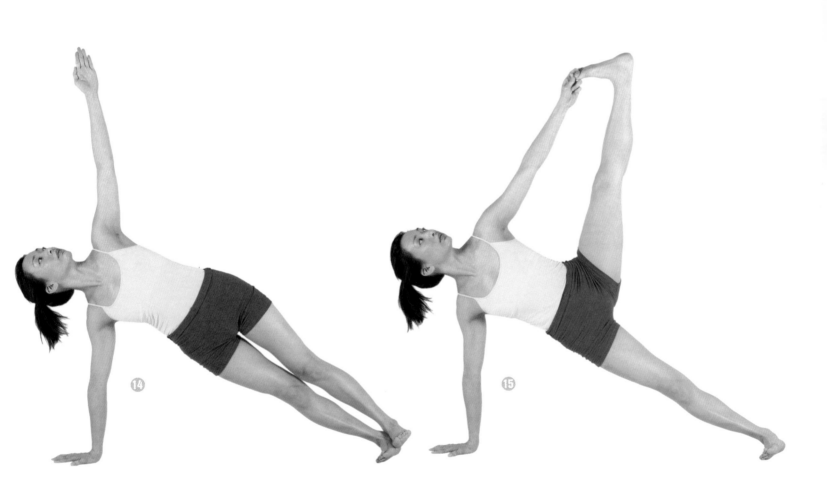

Patricia Walden
Revolved Head-to-Knee
(Parivrtta Janu Sirsasana)

More than a quarter century ago Patricia Walden found her life's work: the practice and dissemination of Iyengar Yoga. But she makes no bones about her distinctly American entry to the path.

"I was living in San Francisco in 1970, and like a lot of people of my generation I was interested in higher states of consciousness," she says. "I read Aldous Huxley and Alan Watts. I took LSD, and that opened some doors for me. I wanted to keep pursuing that expansion."

Patricia became interested in yoga and took her first class from a San Franciscan who wore a loincloth and went by an Indian name. He fueled her already high expectations. "I really felt that if I did yoga for a month, I would become enlightened," she says. If *samadhi* was not instantaneous, a glimpse of it was. "I felt as though I had come home to something that was very familiar, although I'd never done it before," she says. "I felt full—mental, emotional, spiritual fullness. And that introduction planted the seed for future yoga practice."

Patricia returned to Cambridge, Massachusetts, her hometown, in 1975 and found yoga teachers were few and far between. She began practicing on her own, using Swami Vishnu-devananda's *Illustrated Book of Yoga* as a guide. Then she discovered *Light on Yoga*, by B.K.S. Iyengar. "The poses were awe-inspiring and sometimes scary, and the

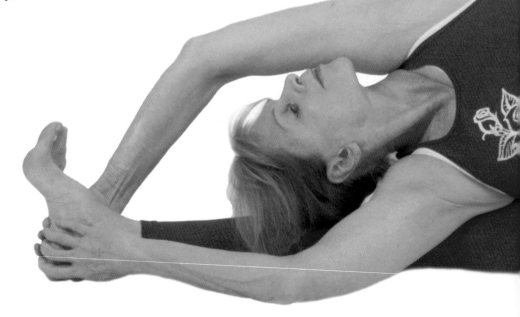

THE YOGA OF THE POSE: "The way it embodies both receptivity and surrender, through the combination of forward-bending, back-bending, and twisting actions. The feeling of space in the chest and torso combined with turning the torso and looking up at the sky brings your being into a receptive state. And because the side body is resting on the thigh, there's also a sense of surrender. Divine presence shoots through the pose, and it has to do with the spine lengthening and your turning the lungs and chest up toward the sky, and how the head and gaze follow that action."

HOW STUDENTS COMMONLY MISS IT: "We need to have our roots firm in the earth in order to feel space and expansion. When someone has tight groins or inflexible hamstrings, they're not able to lengthen their spine and turn freely. If they try to force the hand down to the foot and turn, they lose extension in the legs and freedom in the groin. Also, in seated forward bends people sometimes get uncomfortable with the stillness and think, Oh, I need to go farther; I'm going to no-matter-what get my hands to my feet. That's how people blow their hamstrings and sacroiliac out.

"Another thing: In seated twists people get crabby. Whenever I teach twisting, people feel great when it's finished, but during it, the feeling in the room is not joyful. Twists work on the liver and intestines, and releasing toxins can make people irritable."

HOW TO MAKE SURE YOU CONNECT: "Work with patience! And with props. Start with one leg extended, the other leg bent, and the spine upright, and instead of going all the way down, first turn toward the bent leg and slowly come down. Bend the bottom arm and put it on a bolster or a block if you have to. Extend the top arm but don't try to go for the foot. Forward-bending embodies surrender, but it needs to be cultivated.

"In terms of the twist, there's the whole principle of toning and squeezing organs. Squeezing and then soaking stimulates the intestines so that they function properly. And all this work must be done with the breath. One of the timeless teachings of asana is that we release toxins and negativity through our exhalations."

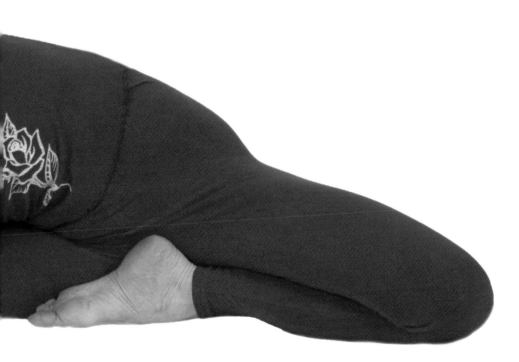

Revolved Head-to-Knee *(Parivrtta Janu Sirsasana)*

Practicing Revolved Head-to-Knee *(Parivrtta Janu Sirsasana)*

1. Begin with the preliminary pose of *Janu Sirsasana* 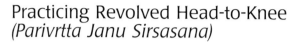. Bend your left knee back to a 90-degree angle and square your torso over your extended leg, which remains active with foot flexed and quadriceps engaged. Bring the sole of your left foot to the upper inner right thigh, or if you're quite flexible take the heel to the inner left groin. Take hold of the right foot or ankle and bow forward, leading with the heart, not with the shoulders and neck ❷.

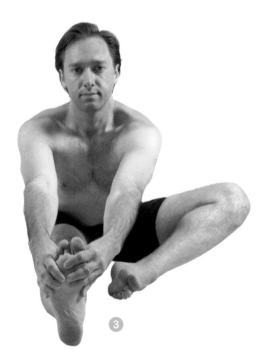

2. In the Kripalu tradition (p. 114) the knee is bent to a far less acute angle, with the foot toward the extended knee, the idea being to square the hips as well as the torso in the pose ❸. Judith Lasater recommends opening up the pose even more by bending the knee less intensely and placing the foot comfortably away from the inner thigh. Try both variations and see how it changes your understanding of *Janu Sirsasana.*

3. If you cannot reach your foot without rounding your shoulders and back, work with a strap ❹ or a towel or sweatshirt (p. 110).

person doing them looked like a creature and not a human. I never thought of actually meeting someone like that."

In fact, those highly advanced postures became the unlikely primer for Patricia's teaching première at the Cambridge Center of Adult Education. "In the first class there were thirty-five people, but I ended up with five people after that. God bless those students. They were finding their way like me, and they liked it! My passion for it spoke to them."

A year later Patricia met B.K.S. Iyengar himself when he came to Wellesley, Massachusetts, as part of his second U.S. teaching tour. "Twenty minutes into class with him I realized I had not a clue as to what I was doing. American yoga teachers in those days would sit in the front of the room with crossed legs and the lights down low, sometimes with their eyes closed, and take people through a series of poses. Guruji stood up on a huge platform with all the lights on. When he started teaching, he came off the platform and walked around and looked at our poses and bodies and said, 'Do this,' and 'Oh, you're not doing that,' and 'Lift more,' and 'Oh, you look depressed.' In just one class I was introduced to my body in a different kind of way, and something changed in me."

"How can you find enlightenment when you can't find your big toe?" B.K.S. Iyengar famously said, and for Patricia the inquiry was profound. "Discipline was a new concept to me at that point," she says. "I was not dealing with life in a practical way. So by talking about how you're standing on your feet, how you're using your legs, how if you want to reach *samadhi*, you had to follow these eight limbs of yoga (p. 56), Guruji began teaching

4. To move into *Parivrtta* (revolved) *Janu Sirsasana,* turn your torso toward the bent knee and take an easy twist there ⑤. Then lean your right shoulder inside the inner right thigh and lay the elbow down with the palm face up. Reach the top arm over your ear. If your shoulder or elbow will not reach the floor, use a block or bolster to make the connection that allows you to open into the pose ⑥.

Revolved Head-to-Knee *(Parivrtta Janu Sirsasana)*

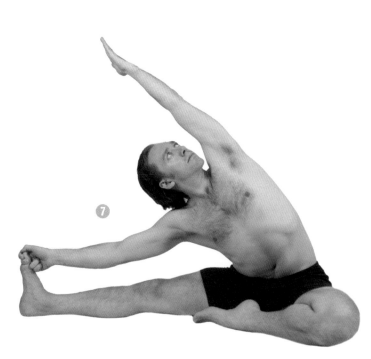

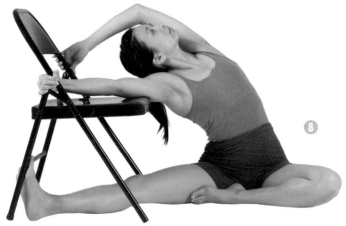

5. As you become ready to move farther into the pose, do whichever of the following allows you to feel length in the right and left side body and openness in the chest. Catch the right big toe in yogic toe lock ⑦; grasp the outer right foot with the left hand and the inner foot with the left hand, as Patricia demonstrates; or use a chair ⑧ to more fully experience the side body reach that is essential to the pose.

me how to live." Iyengar's early Western students often note how he spoke to them through the body, since he did not want to scare people away by making them think yoga is a religion or by talking about God. "He felt that Americans were not ready for that kind of spirituality," Patricia says. "But he wove the philosophy into his teachings."

In 1977 and virtually every year since, Patricia journeyed to Pune, India, to learn more from Iyengar. The first three-week intensive in India "was so hard," she recalls. "Students came from all over the world. After the morning class we would wonder how we were going to walk back to our hotel because our legs were so sore. But there was excitement and joy in it. He was igniting us."

In the mid-1980s Mr. Iyengar's daughter, Geeta, began heading up the inten-

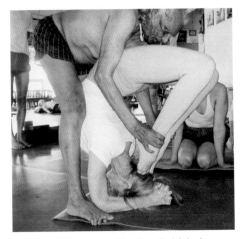

B.K.S. Iyengar adjusting Patricia in Scorpion pose in December 2001.

sives. "She did not like me," Patricia says. "A lot of American women there would dress in Indian clothes, but I wore tight jeans and T-shirts. I was tall and very very thin, probably a little flashy and sexy, and she didn't know what to make of me. Finally she began to understand that just because I presented myself differently didn't mean I wasn't absolutely devoted to the practice."

If B.K.S. Iyengar is what Patricia calls "a poet and scientist and kind of a mad genius," Geeta's pragmatism makes her father's teachings accessible to everyday yoga practitioners—and especially to women, once all but barred from the teachings of yoga. Her influence has combined with Patricia's own experience to formulate novel applications of yoga's benefits throughout the cycles of a woman's life. "For years in this country we've talked openly

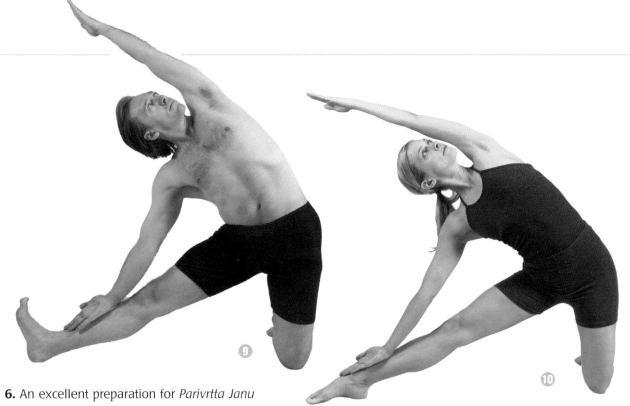

6. An excellent preparation for *Parivrtta Janu Sirsasana* is Gate pose *(Parighasana)*. From a kneeling position, square your hips over your knees as you extend your right leg directly out to the right, with the foot flexed **9** or pointed **10**. Lay the right hand palm face up on the right leg and lean to the right. Gaze up beyond your left arm and breathe into the expansion in the left and right side body.

about PMS and menstruation, but it is just starting to be acceptable to talk about the transitions of perimenopause and menopause." In the yoga community Patricia is among those shaping the conversation.

Patricia recently closed the B.K.S. Iyengar Center of Greater Boston, which she headed up and taught at for eighteen years. She wants time for her writing projects and teaching engagements that keep her traveling around the world much of the year. "To some people my life must look very boring because I don't do a lot except to teach yoga, practice yoga, and study yoga—but I'm happy in it," she says. "I love what I do."

Yoga in America today continues to surprise her. "To go out into Harvard Square and see people with rolled-up mats under their arms is a wow, because when I started doing yoga, there were no mats. And to see Madison Avenue ads with asanas in them is just amazing. The downside is it's given the yoga practitioner a 'look,' and women pay the price. Fitness has different looks, and it's not all size two.

"Yoga class used to be a safe island, a respite from 'image.' I see people in my classes struggle with perfectionism: 'Oh, I can't drop back from *Tadasana*, so I'm not as good as so-and-so, and as soon as I can, I'll be perfect. . . .' I see that more among Westerners than Indians. Eastern practitioners have history and culture behind them. We don't, so we come at it from a very different point of view. I like to address that in my teachings: What makes us feel full? What makes us feel empty? What is the mind that we're bringing to our yoga practice? Because of course that's what it's about."

But what of the size two jeans-clad young woman who journeyed to Pune and practiced asana till her legs gave out—was there no striving there, no perfectionism at work? "Yeah, but you know what?" Patricia Walden says. "It wasn't just that we were striving. We were waking up."

UNDERSTANDING PROPS

The Iyengar tradition has been dubbed "furniture yoga" because of its extensive use of props to enhance the depth and comprehension of the asanas. But Patricia Walden's colleague Mary Dunn emphasizes that these tools are most valuable "not as a crutch to prop you up, but as something that teaches you to let go." If you take yoga class at a gym or community center that does not provide yoga props, purchase them on your own (see Resources Guide) and try using them in class. If you're practicing at home and do not have blocks or straps, use a phone book as a block and a towel or any long, sturdy piece of fabric as a strap. Discover how props can free your body as you work to liberate your mind.

BLOCKS: If a body part does not reach the floor as desired in a pose, raise the floor to meet it by using a block or "brick," as they're sometimes called ❶. These rectangular forms made of Styrofoam or wood offer three levels of support. Turn the block on its smallest edge for the highest prop ❷, on its thinnest side for the second highest ❸, and on its broadest side for the least height ❹. Use the lowest height that allows you to expand fully in the pose.

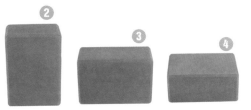

STRAPS: Woven yoga straps or ties can extend the length of your arms and legs ❺. They can keep in place body parts that want to slip away ❻ and offer resistance for instances of overstretched or hyperflexible limbs.

BOLSTERS AND BLANKETS:
Bolsters and folded or rolled blankets
are excellent for making seated poses
steady and comfortable ⑦. They are also
particularly effective for restorative
poses ⑧.

⑧

CHAIRS: An ordinary folding chair can be a
useful tool for backbending ⑨, side bending
(see Step 5), or for restorative work to even out
the pelvis and sacroiliac area ⑩.

⑨

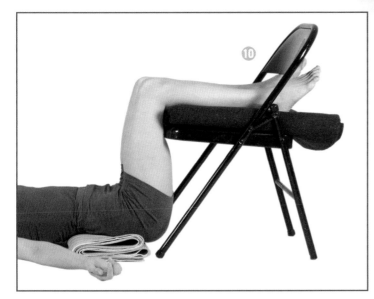

⑩

⑪

THE WALL: Walls offer firm
resistance and support for
experiments with gravity,
stretching, twisting, and
inversions. Examples are
sprinkled throughout the
book, with the simplest—the
Wall Lean—pictured here ⑪.

Stephen Cope
Half Lord of the Fishes
(Ardha Matsyendrasana)

Stephen Cope has a résumé that makes you want to bury your own, or rewrite it. En route to becoming a psychotherapist, he spent a year studying a primitive fishing village in Colombia as part of his undergraduate work in anthropology. He then danced professionally with the Minnesota Dance Theater, after a stint as a scholarship student at the Jacob's Pillow Dance Festival in Lee, Massachusetts. A pianist since childhood, he served as an accompanist at the Boston Conservatory of Music dance department. And he was halfway to earning a master's degree at the Episcopal Divinity School in Boston when he decided that his real interest lay in the psychology of spiritual growth.

Stephen's decision to become a therapist was driven by his desire to heal himself from what he calls "ridiculous family-induced neurosis of the high-WASP kind." He grew up in the storybook town of Wooster, Ohio, where his father was a historian and a dean of Wooster College. Stephen excelled, as expected, in everything from scholastics to sports to religious studies. The town was also home to a group of retired Presbyterian missionaries, several of whom unwittingly gave him his first lesson in yoga philosophy.

"Every Sunday one of the missionaries would come to teach us Sunday school," he recalls. "Three in particular stood out. Dr. and Mrs. Wright had spent their lives in India 'ministering' to the Hindus"—which meant converting them, Stephen notes—"and the experience had imbued them with an aura of wisdom and mystery. They loved to sing, and even while pounding out a hymn like 'Onward Christian Soldiers,' a sense of grace permeated the theology of these people, a sense that we were already saved.

"Every now and then another character would show up to teach: Dr. Wilson, a formal, stern, intellectual man whose approach was so different that I wondered how this could be the same religion. He was all about becoming perfect like Jesus, which we children definitely were not. For Dr. Wilson hell was a very real thing, and he wanted to make it as real for us as it was for him."

So, early on, Stephen perceived two fundamentally opposite views on spirituality: One said we are already okay; the other, that we have our work cut out for us. When as a graduate student in psychotherapy at Boston University he discovered the centering practice of

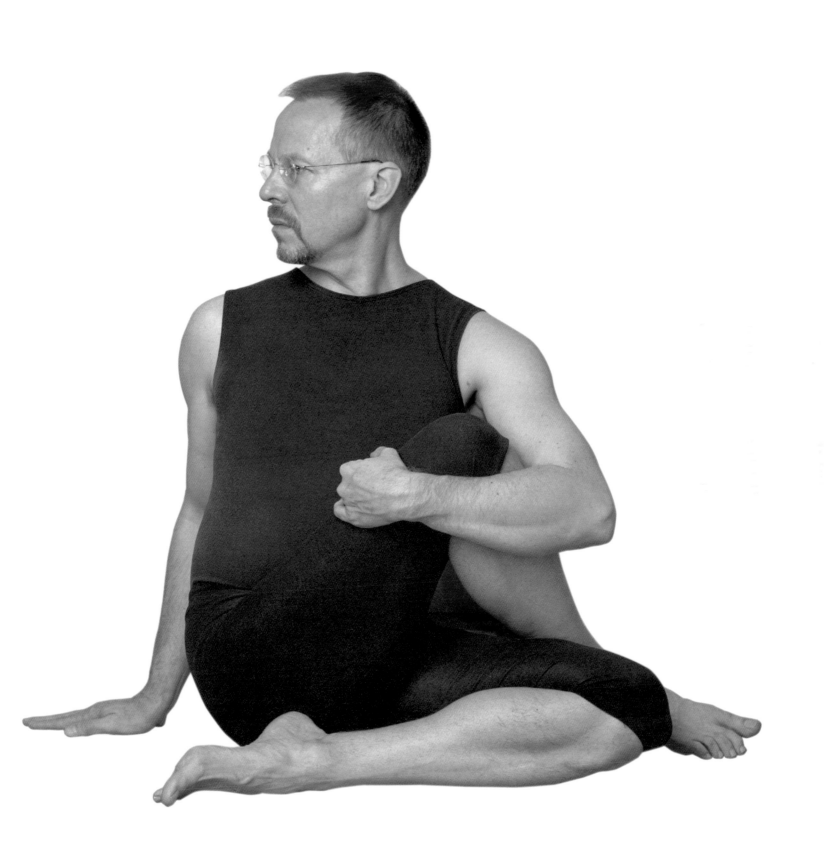

meditation, he figured the dichotomy was finally over. (He later realized it was not. "These two poles seem archetypal in contemplative practice as well," he says, "and they saturate even Eastern thought.")

Stephen had happened upon one of the centers that the Tibetan meditation master Chögyam Trungpa Rinpoche established in the United States and Canada to teach meditation as a tool for everyday living. That application integrated naturally with his study and practice of psychotherapy. But another lesson in opposites occurred when he interviewed for a position at a Boston hospital in the 1970s. During the interview, Stephen stressed the relevance of the meditative state to patient care. "I got ushered out of that office fast," he says.

Twelve years into his practice as a therapist and as a Buddhist, Stephen fell in love with yoga—on his first weekend retreat at Kripalu Center for Yoga and Health, in Lenox, Massachusetts in 1987. "Kripalu Yoga is so dancelike it made me just wild with happiness," he says. "The teacher was tall, beautiful, elegant, and she taught this powerful two-hour class that left me in some kind of altered state." The weekend he was there, the ashram's guru, Amrit

---

THE TALE OF MATSYENDRA

The pose *Matsyendrasana* is dedicated to Matsyendra, the Lord of the Fishes, whom the fifteenth-century text the *Hatha Yoga Pradipika* names as a founder of hatha yoga. The story has it that Lord Siva took his consort, Parvati, to a distant island, where he initiated her into the mysteries of yoga. While he taught her, a lonely fish lay in the waters just off the island, completely still and in a deep state of concentration. So Siva inadvertently taught the fish yoga as well, and when he realized this, he sprinkled it with holy water, at which point the fish realized his divine form. As Matsyendra, he then went on to teach the practices of yoga to the world.

Desai chanced to be there, too. And on that particular Saturday, Gurudev, as his devotees called him, was offering *vandana,* a ceremony in which disciples would receive his blessings and kiss his feet, in the Indian tradition. "I did not believe in this guy and thought the whole thing was kind of silly," Stephen says. "But like a good Protestant at an altar call, I went up anyway. And he actually zapped me. At this point I had never heard the word *Shakti,* but I literally felt energy up and down my spine, and for three days I was blissful."

Stephen took home every video he could buy in the Kripalu Shop and began a regular asana practice that instantly deepened his meditation practice. More and more frequently, he found himself at Kripalu, where he had glimpsed the possibility of a freedom from suffering that did not exist in the psychotherapeutic modality. "It is said, and I believe it's so, that the primary pathology of our culture is the pathology of narcissism," Stephen says. "It was becoming clear to me that what happens in therapy often just continues our narcissistic attachment to the stories of 'me' and 'mine'— the very stories yoga and meditation work to break down." So he took a sabbatical to try to put these two rivers of his life together. Within a year he had shut down his practice in Boston and become a Kripalu resident and yoga teacher. And he had begun an ongoing dialogue with Amrit Desai, whose interest in the psychology of yoga matched his own.

Amrit Desai had come to America in 1960 as an art student, no small feat for the son of a village shopkeeper in the Indian state of Gujarat. Two influences combined to create the willpower that got him here: yoga, as taught to him by his guru, Swami Kripalvananda, and Dale Carnegie's *How to Win Friends and Influence People,* a translated copy of which was given to him at an impressionable age. Calling on both those resources, Desai found great success teaching yoga in America.

The message Desai delivered was highly

attractive to American practitioners. By 1972 he had established an ashram in Sumneytown, Pennsylvania, and had begun teaching Kripalu Yoga, named after his own guru. Kripalu Yoga is rooted in the tradition of Tantra, which at its essence embraces the jollier of the two world-views Stephen discovered as a young boy. Desai's approach to the lineage began with the restraints and observances of the *Yoga Sutras* (p. 56) and blossomed into the Sahaj, or spontaneous yoga, perfected by Swami Kripalu, who had demonstrated to him that the deep inner absorption of meditation can occur within the flow of yoga postures. So in the Kripalu tradition formal sitting and meditation-in-motion are seen as equally valid, complementary practices.

In 1983 Desai moved his Kripalu Ashram to the picturesque town of Lenox, Massachusetts. There he bought what Stephen refers to as a "laughably ugly" brick building that had been constructed to serve as a five-hundred-bed Jesuit monastery. (The grounds, however, designed by Frederick Law Olmsted for a former estate, are extraordinarily beautiful.) By the time Stephen arrived, Desai rarely taught asana per se, but two or three times a year would practice Sahaj Yoga before gatherings of hundreds. "It wasn't so much a demonstration as his own in-the-moment sur-

THE YOGA OF THE POSE: "The sense of absorption the twist provides. *Ardha Matsyendrasana* evokes the same state of inner stillness and concentration Matsyendra dropped into while listening to Siva. I'm not even sure why that happens physiologically, but I know that it certainly does. It also strengthens the connections between the left and right sides of the brain and creates a highly integrated mental state—just as many forms of *pranayama* do.

"I love the contrapuntal nature of the pose— the energy going down to the sitting bones and up the spine at the same time. Fish combine opposing forces into powerful, sleek forward movement, and so does this pose, which gives flexibility to the back, hips, and neck. By squeezing the core of the body, it massages most of the internal organs, especially the digestive tract and the kidneys, and so stimulates digestion and absorption. Some experts say it is excellent for prostate and bladder problems."

HOW STUDENTS COMMONLY MISS IT:
"Students tend to get very rigid in twists, which blocks the energy of the posture. Another mistake people make is to begin the twist from the top of the body—sometimes even in the cervical spine and shoulders.

"The pose must not be collapsed; that's another potential problem. The energy needs to move up the spine in a wave, and that can't happen unless length and lift are maintained through the torso, from the sitting bones to the crown of the head."

HOW TO MAKE SURE YOU CONNECT: "First of all, relax and let the breath saturate the pose. Feel the wave of breath and find a way to connect that with the wave of the twist, which should start as deep in the basement as possible. Visualize the twist originating at the base of the spine, even though very little will move that deep in the body; that's just an energetic movement. But you should feel and think of the actual movement beginning at the navel. Everything else moves in sequence after that, coordinated with breath. Since the twist happens around that energy line, keep the spine long to accommodate it.

"The structure of the posture relaxes a bit on the inhale and deepens a little more on each exhale. This is where the Fish movement comes in. The whole thing breathes! There is the subtlest movement, and it's all about opposition—yet the opposites do not fight but rather balance each other as they flow together seamlessly into resolution."

render to the energy in his body. This was true asana, and his level of concentration drew in the minds of everyone in the room.

"Yoga is not just about movement; it's about the quality of attention we bring to the movement," Stephen says. "I don't think that is fully understood in the West, where the prevailing notion is that yoga is about purifying the body to create a channel for energy. The truth is that energy follows awareness. To make the body a channel of energy, you have to create deeply concentrated states of mind and of focus"—which, of course, had been Stephen's aim from the start.

In 1993 he hosted Kripalu's first major conference, and its subject—psychotherapy and spirituality—proved revolutionary for the ashram. For a start, a panel of outside experts—the renowned therapists Marion Woodman, Jacqueline Small,

Daniel Goleman, Thomas Yeoman, and Sylvia Boorstein—sat up front, while the guru sat at the side of the room. Then, following much discourse on the concept of exposing the "shadow" or disavowed aspects of ourselves, Amrit Desai got up and acknowledged he had one of his own. The specifics of that shadow, which included sexual transgressions in a community built on *bramacharya*, or celibacy, would not come to light for another half year.

And when it did, in October 1994, everything fell apart. "It was chaos," Stephen recalls. "There was a dramatic moment where people attacked the guru's throne and the pictures and icons of the lineage were smashed." Stephen's long experience with psychoanalytic thinking did surprisingly little to mitigate his own shock. But it created a crystalline observation about why things happened as

Practicing Half Lord of the Fishes *(Ardha Matsyendrasana)*

1. To move into *Ardha Matsyendrasana* Kripalu-style, bend your right knee and place your right foot outside your extended left leg at or above the level of the knee. Use your left arm to hug your right knee into your chest, and lengthen your right arm straight ahead ❶.

2. Follow your thumb with your gaze as you inhale and circle your right arm out to the right ❷ and back behind you ❸. Exhale as you place the palm on the floor ❹. You may also bend the left knee and slide your left foot near your right buttock ❺, but not if it causes your right sitting bone to lift off the floor. Remaining grounded through both sitting bones is essential to the posture.

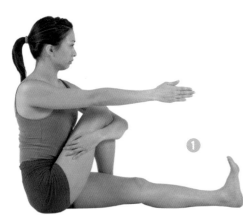

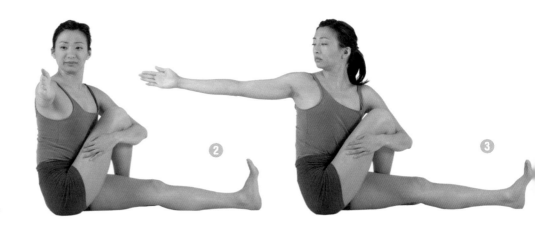

they did—for the community, for himself, and for Desai, the man whose teachings he had valued so highly.

"In the initial transmission of yoga to the West, particular practices were lifted out of a very rich cultural relational surround," Stephen says. "We have received fragments of practice—*pranayama,* meditation, postures—without the context, preliminary practices, and ethical and lifestyle practices to support them." That deficiency, he says, combined with the profound need for belonging that he sees as endemic to modern American society, can lead to an idealization of spiritual teachers that allows for *avidya,* or misperception—for all concerned.

"The human capacity for denial is huge," he says. "This is one of the things that drives me crazy about spiritual life. We think our lovely spiritual projects are what it's really about, and we completely ignore the reality of what's in the basement that also drives our lives. And without inquiring into what it is that is exiled and unconscious, we will remain unaware of our deepest motivations, and our lives will almost always be undermined.

"Carl Jung said that to find out who we are, we have to stay attuned to the voices of our unconscious, and if we don't, our unconscious will find us. Our soul will find a way of engineering it so we hear these messages. Whenever we seem to be brought down by some alien force, it is very often just an exiled part of the Self trying to find its way back into awareness."

In the end, Desai's departure wound up making Kripalu Center a nonsectarian retreat for spiritual seekers of every stripe—due in no small part to Stephen Cope's contagious fascination with yoga's subtle truths. He retains perspective on and beyond the calm view from the Berkshires mountaintop home of what remains the nation's largest yoga center. And he continues to host state-of-the-state-of-yoga conferences that sound the depths of where America's leading teachers are taking the practice. His own journey remains among the most interesting.

Now, about that journey: Is Stephen already there, or is there still a long way to go? "The deepest paradox in spiritual practice is that you have to hold two contrasting views at the same time," he says. "You have to hold that we are all saved and there is nothing we need to do to make that happen. At the same time, the way we live every moment has everything to do with the possibility of enlightenment. So my answer is, if you get stuck on one side or the other, you're in trouble."

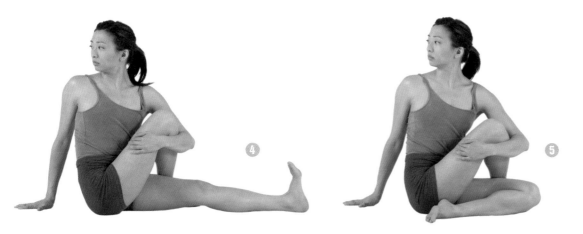

Half Lord of the Fishes *(Ardha Matsyendrasana)*

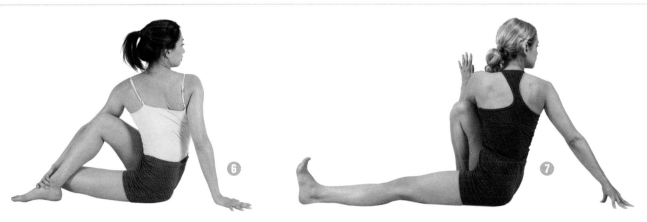

3. The Sivananda Half Spinal Twist ⑥ uses the left arm as a lever to deepen the twist in the mid and upper back. In this variation, press your left arm outside your right knee and take hold of your left ankle with your left hand. Whichever variation you're doing, use the hold on or pressure against your bent knee to lift your sternum as you inhale, then draw the navel to the spine and extend through the crown of the head as you subtly deepen the twist as you exhale.

4. Although the Half Spinal Twist, *Ardha Matsyendrasana,* is included in virtually every style of yoga, Judith Lasater eschews this posture in favor of variations of *Marichyasana III* ⑦. "For most Westerners and especially for most women, *Ardha Matsyendrasana* is a recipe for damaging the sacroiliac joint," she says. "The male sacroiliac joint is structurally much more stable than the female one, so if you're a thin Indian man with a narrow skeleton, then it's not such a problem. But I've worked with hundreds of people with sacroiliac pain that goes away when I move them out of *Ardha Matsyendrasana* and into *Marichyasana III.*"

To take this kinder, gentler twist, bend your right knee and plant your right foot directly in front of your right sitting bone, leaving four to six inches between your right foot and inner left thigh. Inhale your left arm up to the ceiling, and as you exhale, hook your left elbow outside your right thigh and twist to the right, looking out over your right shoulder.

5. Stephen Cope often teaches *Ardha Matsyendrasana* as part of what he calls a "nice, dancelike" posture flow. To begin, draw your right knee back 90 degrees and bow forward over your extended left leg in *Janu Sirsanana* ⑧. After five breaths, sit up, place your right foot outside your left knee, and twist to the right in *Ardha Matsyendrasana* ⑨. Then open your right knee out to the right again, and lift into what Kripalu calls Half-Circle pose, or *Ardha Mandalasana* ⑩, by bringing your right palm to the floor a few inches behind your right buttock, with the fingertips pointing away. Push into your right palm and knee as you inhale and lift the hips and left leg up, sweeping the left hand across the body and up over your ear. Move the hipbones forward, lengthening the left leg and pressing the sole of the left foot into the floor. Breathe deeply into the expansion.

SELF-ANALYSIS: YOGA AND PSYCHOTHERAPY

"Psychologists must not only have a thorough knowledge of the Western science of psychology, but should combine it with Patanjali's Raja Yoga and with spirituality. They will be better able to understand the workings of the mind. Then they will be of more service to the world."

—Swami Sivananda, *Conquest of the Mind*

That regular asana practice promotes healthy bodies and minds is hardly news to yoga practitioners. But as drug manufacturers race to market antidotes for the increasingly common malaise of depression, yoga's psychotherapeutic aspects are being recognized by a nation that is coming to embrace all forms of what is called complementary medicine.

The reasons are clear to longtime yogis and psychotherapists Stephen Cope and Richard Miller. "Depressed people tend to collapse in on themselves, and yoga, with its exploration of opposites, treats the condition in a variety of ways," Richard says. "In asana practice, the body closes and opens, giving people a sense of control they can feel right away. And the moment they come into a yoga class, they're also in community." He stresses the importance of *pranayama* in revitalizing the soul. "One of the first things that contracts in the body is the diaphragm, creating upper respiratory, shallow breathing and a whole host of secondary problems that create an inner environment that breeds further depression. So *Kapalabhati* [p. 186] is a powerful intervention."

In a psychoanalytic climate where biology now holds the fore, "the interesting thing about yoga is that it acts on both the biological, brain chemical aspect while employing a whole philosophy and psychology that addresses behavior motivation," Stephen Cope says. "The very best psychotherapy requires the therapist to be in a state similar to what yogis call the Witness. Freud described this state as one of 'evenly hovering attention,' and the great English psychoanalyst W. R. Bion famously said that the therapist must suspend both memory and desire—

in other words, let go of the past and the future and be fully present in the moment. When the therapist is abiding in the Witness state, the patient's own witness consciousness is awakened. And when a yoga teacher is fully present in that consciousness, it helps to awaken the students' witness. It's profound when it happens, and it happens all the time in good yoga classes."

Francesca Nadalini, a psychotherapist in northern New Jersey, has observed that to be true even though she does not practice yoga herself. Through patients who do, she began to note how effective the combination of yoga and psychotherapy can be. "When one of my patients entered therapy, he simply could not function," she recalls. "He was rolled up in a ball on the floor sobbing. So he was put on medication, but he also took up yoga on his own. It was clear that the yoga helped him deal with the emotional work, the anxiety and fear that come up with psychoanalysis. Patients who do in-depth work get physical symptoms they can't actually quantify, and I can see it—if they do yoga and they work their breath, they can deal with symptoms so much better."

For another patient, "a woman with a shallow, raggedy breathing pattern who has been told she doesn't speak up enough," Dr. Nadalani recommended the aid of a *pranayama* teacher. "Breath is the contact with life from the minute we're born. You take that first breath reluctantly, and it mediates the world for you. A person who is not breathing fully is not able to live fully; it's like living at half-mast. And it can be corrected; that's the beauty of it. Breathing is the mind-body connection, which is essential to psychotherapy."

Dr. Nadalini continues to recommend yoga to her patients and plans to begin lessons herself. Her mentor, Joseph Masterson of the Masterson Institute for Psychoanalytic Psychotherapy in New York, "always said the therapist ought to be guardian of the real Self." From his ashram in Rishikesh, India, sixty years ago, Swami Sivananda announced the same conclusion.

Emmy Cleaves

Camel
(Ustrasana)

Emmy Cleaves took her first yoga class in 1950 from a Hindu in Beverly Hills. As a young war refugee from Latvia, her trajectory to that tony locale had been at least as unlikely as his. So when she later became a convert to the methodology of another Hindu in Beverly Hills—Bikram Choudhury—the universality of the teachings remained clear to her. "There's only one kind of yoga," she says. "There are just different paths to it because we are such a myriad of people. We are all God's experiment of one."

Emmy was a young girl when she and her mother fled their hometown of Riga, Latvia, during the Stalinist army's second advance on the tiny country at the start of World War II. "We tried to escape to Sweden but were intercepted by German patrol boats," she says. "We wound up in a labor concentration camp." Emmy nearly died at Danzig, where the Nazis used Jews, Russians, "any conceivable configuration of people," to fuel their war machine. "The food was seventy-five percent sawdust mixed with twenty-five percent flour. My stomach stopped functioning. It was all jammed up with sawdust."

When the Eastern front advanced on Danzig, the camp disintegrated, and Emmy, separated from her mother, was shipped off to Denmark, then back to Germany, and finally to the United States. "Refugees were sent wherever somebody would take them, and I was very lucky that a family in Grand Rapids, Michigan, sponsored me, enabling me to come to America." In her late teens, with no money and no job, she found her way to the YWCA in Chicago, where she was told she could stay if she worked the front desk. "And I did— with my terrible broken English." She learned the language, got a better job, and became reunited with and married to a fellow refugee, with whom she moved to California.

Emmy was a successful businesswoman in Los Angeles by the time she attended that

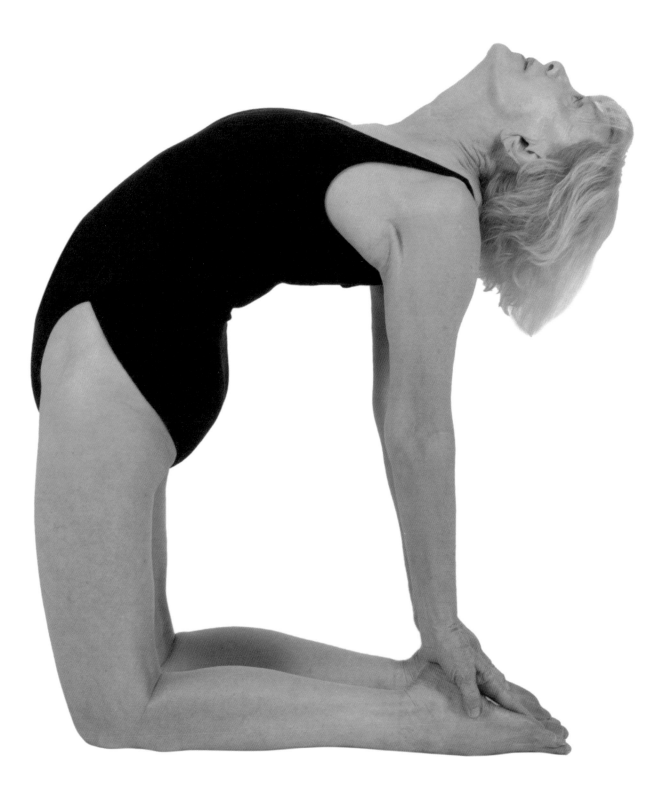

first yoga class. She had been pestering her jazz dance teacher for more of the slow stretching exercises he taught as warm-ups, so he told her to do yoga—the first time she had heard the word. "I became completely fascinated with the subject," she says. For her, as for most practitioners, the initial attraction was physical. "But when I started learning the philosophy, it seemed like, yes, that's exactly it; that's the truth," she recalls, "the ethics and morality that my mother had taught me. I had always sensed that we're not just a quantum mechanical body, that we're really multidimensional beings, and that the body is just a denser form of the many interactive energy fields. So it all resonated completely with my state of mind."

Emmy began reading books and practicing on her own. She got initiated in Maharishi Mahesh Yogi's Transcendental Meditation technique, which cured her of the migraine headaches she had suffered since childhood. For the next two decades she sampled the relatively limited smorgasbord of yoga offerings then available in Los Angeles. "I would try a class here, at the Y, somewhere else—but I never was impelled to stay,

THE YOGA OF THE POSE: "The Camel opens you up on every level. As the posture changes the structure and chemistry of the body, it changes feelings and behavior. The physical manipulation causes a shift in your mental attitude, and as your relationship with yourself improves, so does your relationship with others.

"On a physical plane, it gives your spine, lungs, and heart more room. The tissue of the lungs takes only about ten percent of the ribcage space; it's mostly air and blood. So the more space you make for air and blood, the more it can circulate in the heart and lungs, the healthier you're going to be. And the pulling up and out of your hips, opening the front part of the body, and just saying 'Here I am'—that is what Camel is about to me."

HOW STUDENTS COMMONLY MISS IT: "If they're reluctant to do it because they don't want to go there. Psychologically it's a very threatening posture to a lot of people. You see, we all protect our heart. There's a lot of implosion and pulling in around it. And the more you scrunch everything in, the less oxygen you get, because you've compressed the lower part of the lungs, which has the most oxygen receptors. The person who walks around with a hunched back, whose shoulders are all pulled over the sternum, is pulled in and protected—that manifests not only on a physical level.

"So when someone like that tries to do Camel, they tend to sink back into the arms instead of keeping the weight forward in the pelvis and knees. They collapse backward and miss all of this wonderful expansive feeling."

HOW TO MAKE SURE YOU CONNECT: "When you're willing and ready to start opening your heart, that's when the Camel comes into its full force. The pose gives you a chance to do that because you're working to some degree with gravity by going back, grabbing your heels with your hands, and then pushing against gravity. And then you get this internal dimension of moving the sternum up and out of the ribcage and more open to the ceiling. And you get in touch with the fact that there is more room available to you.

"So keep your weight forward in the hips and knees and open the chest by lifting the sternum. Use your hands on your hips and buttocks to help push yourself forward until eventually you go back, testing yourself, getting deeper into it. And as you do repetitions of that"—the Bikram method involves two sets per asana—"you start getting looser. The body's very plastic. You're not sentenced to being in whatever position you think you're going to be stuck in."

Practicing Camel (Ustrasana)

1. Kneel with your knees hip-width apart, placing a folded mat or blanket under the knees and shins if this is uncomfortable. Tuck your toes under and place your hands on your lower back. Keep the hips directly over the knees as you open across the collarbones and lift the sternum toward the ceiling ❶. From here, see if it is possible for you to lower your right hand to your right heel and your left hand to your left heel, as Emmy is demonstrating. Keeping your toes tucked under makes it easier to reach your heels. But if you cannot reach, continue to lift your heart with your hands on your back, and breathe ease across the collarbones. "What goes on in your brain is as important as what goes on in your body," Emmy says. "It's always mind-body, body-mind. There is no division."

2. If you experience fear in Camel, try taking the same basic shape from a more stable foundation, suggests Richard Miller. Sit on your heels in Thunderbolt pose, or *Vajrasana*, interlace your fingers behind your back, and press the knuckles to the floor behind you, keeping your chest over your hips ❷. Separate your hands and prop yourself up on your fingertips if bringing your fist down makes you recline. Or become more accustomed to opening your chest in Cobra ❸ "until you have a sense of relaxation and control, and then go deeper into it with the sense of being able to meet your fear without being overwhelmed by it," Richard says. "If you're overwhelmed, you'll just be retraumatized."

3. The Locust *(Salabhasana)* is another good preparation for Camel. Lie on your abdomen with your arms alongside your body. On an inhale lift everything off the floor but your belly and the backs of your hands ❹. Length is more important than lift here, so don't bend your knees or crane your neck to bring yourself up higher. Stay for five strong, slow breaths and release.

4. If you are quite comfortable in Camel, try lowering the crown of your head toward the floor ❺. Walk your hands toward the backs of your knees, and breathe into the expansion across your chest as you gaze beyond the tip of your nose or between your brows. "I sometimes let my eyes go way up or way down," Erich Schiffman says. "My *drishti* [gaze] is on the experience of the moment."

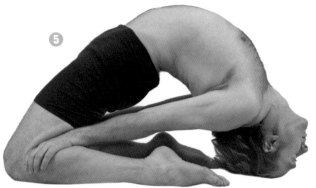

because internally I didn't connect with anyone," she says. "The teacher has to resonate on some other level than just 'Put your legs here' and 'do this' and 'stretch that.'"

Then, at thirty-five, Emmy nearly died again—this time from a brain hemorrhage, which is what had killed her father back in Latvia. Emmy survived and recovered, as only twenty percent of cerebral aneurysm sufferers do. But the experience changed her forever. "A life-threatening event like that makes you wonder what the purpose is of your survival. Why are you alive? Why didn't you die?" Emmy's search for answers created cata-

clysmic upheavals in her life. She gave up being a businesswoman. She divorced her first husband. And she began exploring meditation and yoga much more seriously.

In 1973 Emmy went to a demonstration given by a twenty-six-year-old yogi by the name of Bikram Choudhury. "His group consisted of maybe ten people—all ages and shapes, including a couple of kids. I was fascinated by the energy and precision of his demonstration." At the end of the presentation Bikram jumped off the stage, walked across the room, and stuck his card in her hand. "Tomorrow. You come. My school," he said. She did.

As chance had it, in the preceding weeks Emmy had been reading *Autobiography of a Yogi*, by Paramahansa Yogananda, whose brother Bishnu Ghosh had been Bikram's guru throughout his childhood in Calcutta. Ghosh, a master of yoga's physical practices, trained young Bikram to compete in the National India Yoga Competition, which Bikram won at age eleven and for the next three years. At Ghosh's behest Bikram set off to teach in the West, making his way from Japan to Hawaii to San Francisco and finally to Beverly Hills, where he began reteaching Emmy Cleaves everything she had ever learned.

"We argued. We really argued," Emmy says. "I had done yoga for a long time, none of it the way he demanded it be done." Bikram's methodology involves a basic series of twenty-six poses practiced in a 105-degree brightly lit mirror-lined room with indoor-outdoor carpeting— the very antithesis of the typical yoga studio. The asanas look different too. "I would go into the Cobra doing everything right," Emmy says, "and he would say, 'No, that's not the way. The posture's not the object; your body is the object.' I

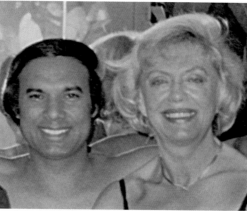

Emmy with her teacher, Bikram Choudhury, at his school in Beverly Hills, California in 1975.

began getting very frustrated. And that heat! I said, 'Bikram, if you'd turn down the stupid heat, this room would be much more full.' He said, 'An empty barn is better than a barn full of naughty cows.'"

Emmy had had enough. "It was upsetting my whole equilibrium," she says. Her friend Barbara Brown, a pioneer in the development and popularization of biofeedback, was taking a trip to India to tour medical research centers, and Emmy joined her. Among the facilities she investigated was a medical clinic in Tirupati, in southern India, where yoga was being used to treat diabetes and

asthma. "Lo and behold, they did the individual postures Bikram's way," Emmy says. "I visited three or four other research centers that did the poses his way, too, with the same energy, the same demand for precision."

So Emmy went back to Beverly Hills and immersed herself in Bikram's teachings and in the logic of his twenty-six-posture, ninety-minute series. (The advanced series, also an hour and a half long, comprises eighty-four postures.) "The first time you do the twenty-six postures, which cover a normal range of motion for just about anybody, they act as a diagnostic tool," she explains. "Even people with minimal body awareness are able to diagnose their own problem areas. Then with practice, those same postures become therapeutic tools that reeducate your body and heighten the efficiency of its major systems."

Like any well-chosen asana program, Bikram Yoga is intended to tone the endocrine, lymphatic, and digestive systems, increase capillary blood flow, and produce a strong, limber, and comfortable musculoskeletal system. To attain the benefits of this series, though, the sequence of the postures is paramount, which is why Emmy defends Bikram's decision to copyright his method. "If you take the formula for penicillin and leave out one of the ingredients, you no longer have penicillin, right?"

While Emmy became one of Bikram's earliest teachers, she did not enter into a guru-disciple relationship with this man young enough to be her son. "I'm a completely Western woman, and I had no interest in becoming an ersatz Hindu. But Bikram is my teacher, and I'm deeply grateful to him. He instilled a deep passion in me for yoga and for sharing whatever I know about it with others."

Camel *(Ustrasana)*

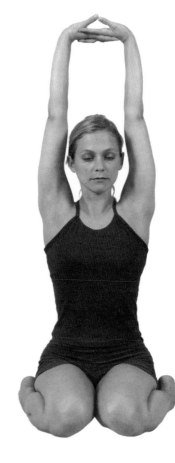

5. After or between practicing Camel, rest in Hero pose *(Virasana).* Separate the shins, roll the calf muscles out and back, and lower your buttocks between your feet, sitting on a rolled-up blanket, towel, or block if your buttocks do not reach the floor ❻. Keep your knees together or at least parallel and take care to align the shins, ankles, and tops of feet. Hero is a recommended seat for meditation or *pranayama.* So quiet yourself here by interlacing your fingers and pressing the palms up to the ceiling ❼. If you can sit easily on the floor, move into *Supta Virasana* ❽, or Fixed Firm pose, as it is known in the Bikram tradition. Lift your tailbone and send it toward your knees, then lie down and breathe into this deep stretch of the quadriceps and iliopsoas muscles in the front of your thighs that prepares the body for deeper backbends like *Urdhva Dhanurasana* (p. 128). After *Virasana,* move into Downward-Facing Dog and stretch your legs all the way down to your heels to open the knee joints ❾.

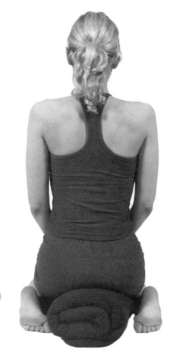

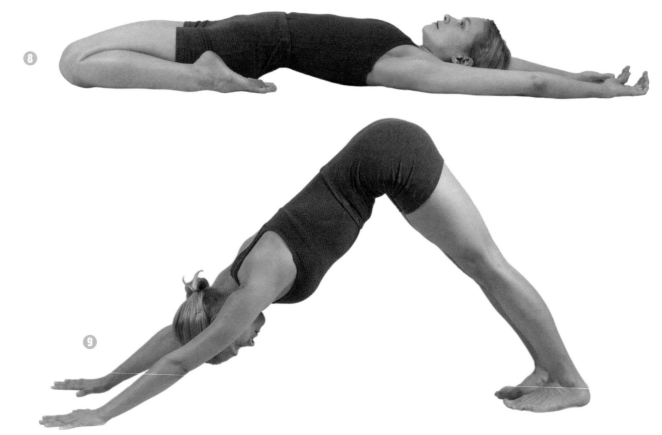

Much attention has been given to Bikram's ostentatious lifestyle and over-the-top teaching style, in which he barks outlandish words of dubious encouragement into his headset microphone while perched atop a makeshift throne in a black Speedo swimsuit and gold jewelry. But that's not how Emmy remembers him. "When Bikram first started being Bikram, he was the gentlest, purest spirit you'd ever want to meet. As students walked in, he would say, 'Well—four dollars; just leave it at the desk.' And you'd be surprised how many rich Beverly Hills people never left a penny and took his towels besides. Now he's at the stage of when in Rome, do as the Romans do. But once in a while I still see the pure being I met, and the rest is just a coat he's wearing—a coat of Rolls-Royces and diamond watches."

The efficacy of Bikram Yoga is made continually apparent to Emmy through the many therapeutic "miracles" she has witnessed in the thirty years she has taught it, with remediation of Type 2 diabetes chief among them. Emmy herself, who had been put on thyroid medication in her thirties and told she'd have to take it for the rest of her life, no longer needed it after she began the practice.

"What gives me such pleasure is that I am able to share this valuable thing, which has so much potential to better people's lives and to heal whatever is not working for them," Emmy says. "That is the ultimate accomplishment of my life and will be to the end of it." The end is not in sight, if genetics has anything to do with it. Emmy's mother, whom Emmy finally found and brought to America in the 1960s, lived to be 102. And that bodes well for anyone looking for a yoga teacher in Beverly Hills.

6. Bow pose, or *Dhanurasana* ⑩, takes Camel on its belly, with the floor as reinforcement against the collapsing action Emmy warns against. Lie down on your abdomen and reach back to take hold of your ankles, shins, or the tops of your feet. Different teachers will instruct you differently, so see what feels best for you as you inhale and kick your feet up and back to lift your chest and thighs. If you cannot reach your feet, keep the arms alongside the body and lift the thighs and chest all you can. Remember to lead with the chest, not the chin, and breathe calmly into the expansion.

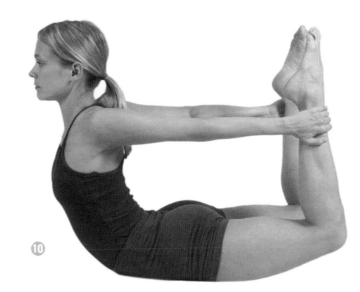

Dharma Mittra
Upward-Facing Bow
(Urdhva Dhanurasana)

Under the loving surveillance of the venerable New York yoga teacher Dharma Mittra, students boldly go where they have never gone before. "Go ahead, try," he commands sweetly in an impossible-to-place accent that sounds like a cross between Bela Lugosi and God. So you go ahead and try whatever logic-defying asana he has just brought to life from his 908-posture Master Yoga Chart (pp. 132–133), the poster he made in 1983 that has become standard decor at American yoga centers. And in Dharma's presence you just may succeed.

Dharma was born and raised in Pirapora, Brazil, a river town named for the fish that migrate there to begin their swim upstream. From the age of thirteen he was "hungry and thirsty to find out what is eternal, what is the truth," he says. His mother's relatives were devout Catholics and Masons with an interest in the occult, so early on, Dharma delved into notions of reincarnation and karma. When he was eighteen, he discovered yoga.

"My younger brother had lots of yoga books, and one day I sneaked into them," Dharma says. "I started reading, and I thought, That's it! I have found it." In an upstream swim of his own, Dharma continued his study throughout the seven years he served in the Brazilian air force. "I was trying, through relaxation, to go beyond the body consciousness, to do some breathing so that the mind is slowed to a point where you go into another state," he says. But he had yet to incorporate the practice of asana.

Then in 1962 his brother, who had moved to New York, sent a letter saying he had found a guru—and that he was the real deal. "So I quit the air force and became a full-time yogi," Dharma says. He scraped together $330 for airfare to New York City, where he shared his brother's Greenwich Village apartment and began studying with Swami Kailashananda, also known as Yogi Gupta. "When I met him, it was just like meeting God," Dharma says. "I could not even look straight at his head."

Yogi Gupta, like many great Indian yoga masters, was born to a family of wealth and privilege. Although he was ordained as Swami Kailashananda and served as an *acharya*, or teacher, at Swami Sivananda's Yoga Vedanta Forest University, he moved on to establish his own order. A lawyer before he renounced the world, Yogi Gupta apparently retained several quite worldly principles, charging seven to eight times the going rate for

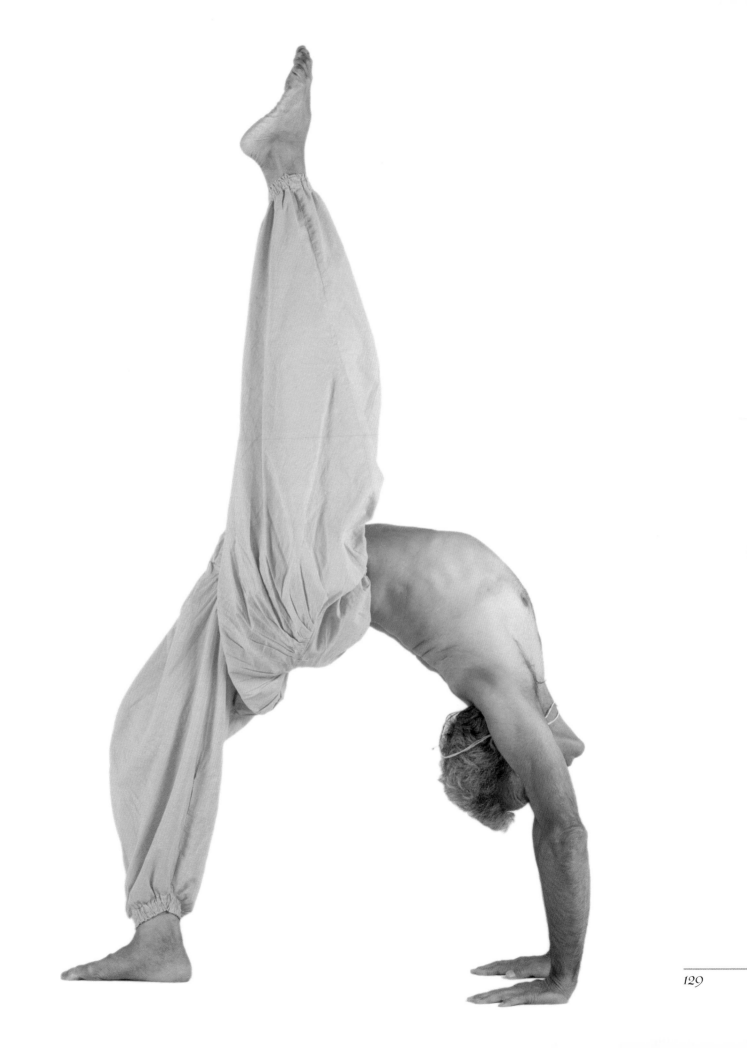

yoga classes. Some portion of the proceeds went to his Kailashananda Mission, the ashram he established on vast acres of family-owned land back in Rishikesh, India, and Western devotees like Dharma were more than happy to contribute.

"I spent all my money with my guru," he says contentedly. "Everything was just for yoga. Some of the classes were thirty-five dollars and some thirty dollars, but if I could pay a million dollars, I would!"

During his first three years in New York, Dharma was earning sixty dollars a week by working overtime as a porter at Manhattan General Hospital, "a hospital for drug addicts. They liked me there because I was very controlled, and they would see me drink my celery juice and eat my sprouts." When he wasn't tending the ward, Dharma was attending yoga class. The solid grounding in asana he gained from his guru deepened his understanding of the discipline immeasurably. "Oh, yes, most definitely," he says, "because it brings flexibility and good health. Also I learned that you must practice one pose for a long time so that you shift consciousness—and then you begin to experience something in meditation."

It is said that in yoga there are four types of students: feeble, average, superior, and supreme. Dharma was clearly among the last group. After three years Yogi Gupta sent him out to teach on his own, renting a space for him at the Hotel San Carlos on 50th Street. "I started teaching there," Dharma says. "I barely could speak English, but gradually I learned, and since 1967 I have been teaching this yoga."

Yoga students in New York tend to find their

THE YOGA OF THE POSE: "It's like an act of adoration to the Lord. So your mental attitude during the pose is very important. You should not expect anything from it. But when your spine is that curved, that flexible, you feel young and healthy. So you may be young, but if you're stiff, you feel old. You may be old, but if you are flexible, you're as healthy as if you're young.

"The Upward Bow is considered a semi-inversion—not a full inversion pose, but a tremendous amount of blood is going down to your brain. When your leg is all the way up, all the blood keeps going down to your head, like in Headstand. You feel actually very good after the pose, because it induces sleep. If you lie down to relax after, you will fall asleep."

HOW STUDENTS COMMONLY MISS IT: "Some people don't have faith, some people do not eat properly, and some people don't practice enough."

HOW TO MAKE SURE YOU CONNECT: "Keep practicing and practicing. If your body is a normal body, if you practice with faith, trying to eat properly—everyone may achieve this. If you want to achieve faster, you get full time in that pose, you achieve it in a few weeks. But if you want to practice less, for lazy people, once a week, twice a week, it sometimes takes years.

"Some people are fortunate. They are born flexible, and they don't have to do any basic poses. But otherwise, there are basic poses they have to practice, like the Bow, the Downward-facing Dog to get your arms moving back, and the Cobra. Then, you have to stay long enough in the pose, breathe normally, and concentrate in the right place. I was instructed by my guru that in *Urdhva Dhanurasana,* you concentrate on the third eye. For advanced students, they must do *asvini-mudra,* the contraction of the anal muscles. That excites your *shakti* and tends to force the vital energy up your spine. Sometimes, when you do it very hard, you feel high.

"The rest of the instruction has to be imparted psychically. It is up to the student to copy the teacher mentally and spiritually."

Practicing Upward-Facing Bow *(Urdhva Dhanurasana)*

1. Begin with Bridge *(Setu Bandhasana)* ①. Lie down on your back, bend your knees, and place your feet parallel and hip distance apart, with your heels close to your sitting bones. Press into your feet, lift your hips, and wriggle your arms under your body one by one, interlacing your fingers and pressing the outer edges of your wrists and upper arms to the floor. Keep your knees pointing straight out over your toes. If your thighs splay out, strap them into parallel alignment or try squeezing a block between them. Extend the tailbone toward your knees and your sternum toward your chin. Rolling the shoulders and upper arms out and under is a prerequisite to opening the chest and shoulder girdle, so if tight shoulders or heavy upper-body musculature prohibit that rotation, use a strap to help maintain it.

2. From Bridge, bend your elbows and place your palms alongside your ears with the fingers pointing toward your feet. As you inhale, lift up onto the top of your head ②. Look at your elbows and draw them toward each other until they are parallel and directly over your wrists.

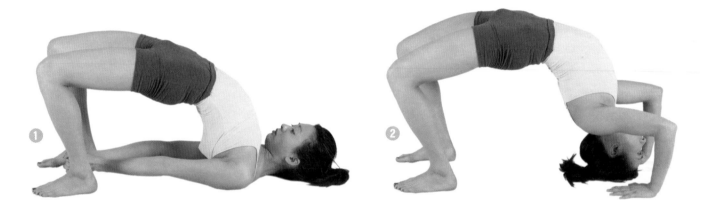

3. Press into your hands and feet and lift up into Upward-Facing Bow ③. To ensure that your feet remain parallel, pigeon-toe them a bit before you come up. As you lengthen the front of the body from sternum to pubic bone, re-create Upward-Facing Dog with your chest and Downward-Facing Dog with your arms. Breathe calmly and deeply in the pose. Backbends, which are said to help us move forward in our lives, stir strong emotions in practitioners new and old. The seasoned yogi learns to watch those feelings come and let them go. But if your body is not yet ready to take the shape, your apprehension may be well founded. "Fears may arise because the mind is trying to strive so hard that the body is actually getting injured," Richard Miller points out. Be patient with yourself as you begin the practice of backbending by practicing the preparatory poses suggested for *Ustrasana* (p. 123).

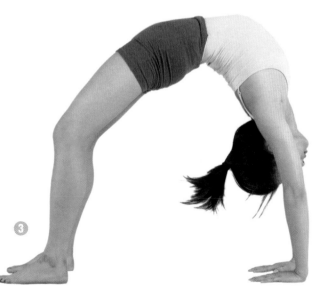

Dharma Mittra's 908-pose Master Yoga Chart. Although most people call *Urdhva Dhanurasana* "Full Wheel," Dharma insists you cannot unless your hands meet your feet, as in asana number 535 (above).

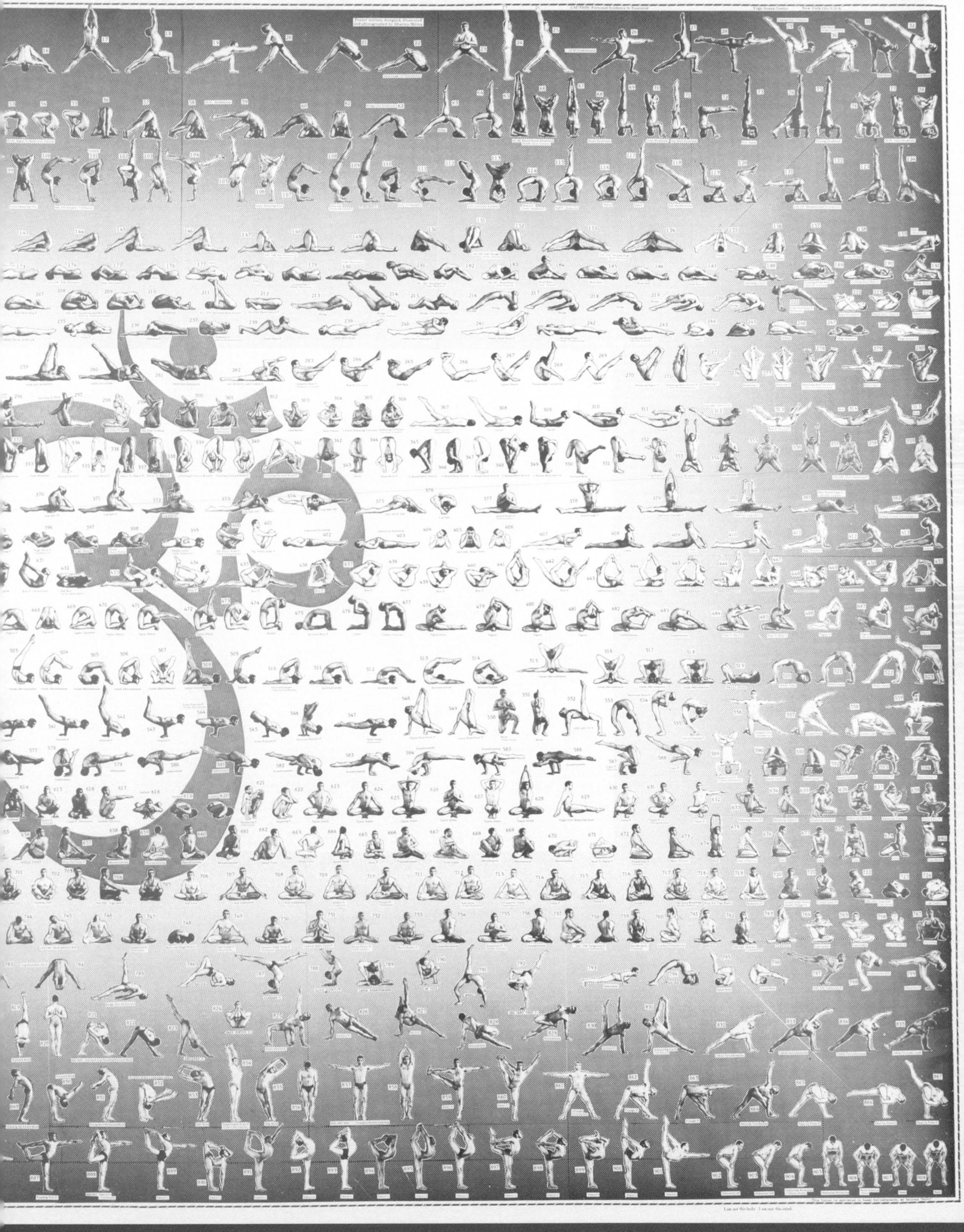

Upward-Facing Bow *(Urdhva Dhanurasana)*

way to Dharma's school, now at 23rd Street and Third Avenue. And since virtually every teacher in town has made the pilgrimage over the years, his influence gets disseminated in interesting ways—as in the case of one student turned teacher from Japan who delivers Sanskrit posture instruction in Brazilian-Japanese–tinged English.

Dharma had been teaching New Yorkers for sixteen years when he decided to create the Master Yoga Chart as an offering to his guru and to yoga aspirants. "We printed 5000 to start and actually almost gave them away; and then, after many years, it became popular," he says. (He has sold upward of 50,000.) To design the poster, Dharma collected yoga books "from every place" and painstakingly photographed himself in some 1300 poses.

"Every day I set the camera about twenty feet away, with a video camera behind it. I had a remote control, and for some poses I had to hold that part in my mouth." He would check the monitor, finesse the angles, squeeze the remote with his teeth, and spit it mightily out of the frame in the five-, four-, or three-second interval before the shutter snapped. ("It was a very old Nikon," he recalls, "and as the project went on, it gave me less and less time.") Dharma worked round the clock to cut out each image, select 908 among them, pin them sequentially on a board, and cut and paste them all over again once they were digitized. The project took three long months.

In 1986 Dharma ended his long years as a *brahmachari,* a celibate who devotes himself to the practice of spiritual disciplines, by marrying a devoted student named Eva Grubler, who he says was extremely flexible and "quiet there like a mouse. When I met Eva I told her the purpose of getting together is to raise children and not to fool around. I told her, 'If you want to be involved with me, we have to go down to City Hall and get married.' " In less than one week the couple took the trip downtown.

Eva and Dharma's son and daughter are now thirteen and twelve, respectively. "It's a wonderful opportunity, to raise these two souls," he says. "We taught them the first step of yoga: *ahimsa.* You don't hurt the animals, you don't step on the ants, you don't be cruel to the dog, you don't do this with the cat. You don't eat meat because of this and that. So they understand a little bit the laws of karma. But you know, I almost can see them gone, the children. In another five years they get married, they go away, they love more their wives and husbands, and they sometimes maybe show up just once a year to borrow some money."

Dharma Mittra (third from left) with his guru, Yogi Gupta, in New York City in 1966.

Dharma no longer practices all 908 poses on his Master Yoga Chart—which has nothing to do with his being in his mid-sixties. "The age is not a problem; every year I notice I am a little more flexible," he says. "The only difference, you just have to take longer to warm up. But since I got married, it's hard planning to practice. Children, distractions, teaching too much—two days away and you forget yourself. But if I really want to achieve a pose, I start practicing that, and in a few more days I can catch it back again."

He is still learning poses. "Every time I have students, they came from another guru, and they have another pose I don't know," he says. "And I am always busy doing workshops here and there in the country, and during those, I attend someone

4. If you are tight and inflexible in the shoulders, chest, and back, try *Urdhva Dhanurasana* with a strap to keep your arms parallel. Prop your hands up on blocks to aid the opening of chest and shoulders 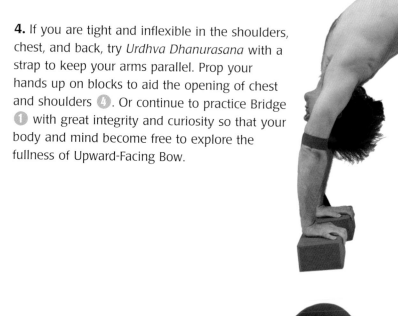. Or continue to practice Bridge ❶ with great integrity and curiosity so that your body and mind become free to explore the fullness of Upward-Facing Bow.

5. Dharma Mittra encourages students to pull their head all the way through their arms in Downward-Facing Dog ❺ as a way of attaining the openness in the shoulders and chest that facilitates Upward-Facing Bow as well as poses like *Eka Pada Rajakapotasana* (p. 151). Crescent Moon pose ❻, from the Sivananda tradition, opens the psoas muscles in the fronts of the thighs, which deepens your ability to curve the spine.

6. After Upward-Facing Bow, position the soles of your feet parallel to the ceiling and reach for their inner or outer edges, pulling your knees toward the floor outside your armpits **7**. This pose, nicknamed Happy Baby or Dead Bug, releases the lower back. Keeping the knees apart in this way is a gentler transition than the common instruction to pull both knees toward your chest.

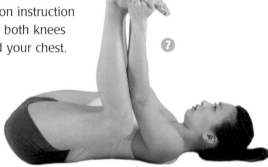

else's class and learn different things. So I keep adding more and more postures." Which raises the question: How many more can there be? "Well, they say the number is infinite," Dharma notes. "As time passes, all the teachers who are in a state of bliss, they usually develop postures. Every year you may notice there are new postures developed by some yogis."

He has been responsible for more than a few. "Well, I don't say me—it's whatever is passing through me. But there are maybe thirty, fifty poses that are very popular today that came to me by intuition and I placed in the posture. But I must say, 'Oh, this is from God. He made that.' And the pose, it's not actually new. It's just variations."

When Dharma was studying with Yogi Gupta,

7. A simple supine twist feels great after backbending. Draw your knees to your chest, square your hips under your shoulders, and drop both knees to the right, gazing out over your left shoulder **8**. You can weigh your left knee down with your right hand to keep it stacked on your right knee.

8. *Paschimottanasana* after backbending brings everything back to neutral. Pull the buttocks flesh back and away so you feel your sitting bones on the floor beneath you. Activate your quadriceps by flexing your feet so strongly your heels lift off the floor **9**. But if your hamstrings are overly flexible, accelerate a gas pedal with the ball of each foot to allow the fronts of the legs to do their part. Take your big toes, your feet, use a strap, or bend your knees to move into a forward bend that feels good to you.

all the other students sat with pen and paper in hand, furiously scribbling notes on his every move. But Dharma just watched. Finally he approached his teacher with concern. "'Yogi Gupta, all I do is copy you.' And he came right up to my nose and said, 'That's it!'"

"You become what you copy," Dharma says. "Let's say you love Mozart. You must copy him and channel his energy; that's how you learn how the fingers move, all the tricks. As you try to copy asana from someone, you come to know by intuition. Everyone who has a spiritual teacher must pretend and copy him mentally, spiritually. And then you start to be like him; you know everything all the time."

It is a dear thing to be singsonged into *Savasana*

by Dharma Mittra. "Now you lay down and rest there like a corpse," he says. "No memories—not any*thing*!" And when you sit back up to close the practice with some meditation and chanting, Dharma reminds you, "To the right of the heart there is a cavity the size of your thumb; that's the location of the spiritual heart. If you want to talk to God, go within. Everything is there.

"The supreme teacher in the heart is the only one," Dharma says. "All the other gurus, they're not the real, real, real, real one. They're just to show you the real guru there in your heart. Both of you work in trying to polish that stone, and gradually it becomes this huge diamond. It turns you into an angel."

9. To do Inclined Plane *(Purvottanasana),* a lovely counterpose to *Paschimottanasana,* come up to sit and place your palms eight to ten inches behind you with your fingers facing your buttocks ⑩. On an inhale press into your hands and feet to lift your hips higher than your knees and your chest higher than your shoulders. Press all ten toes into the floor.

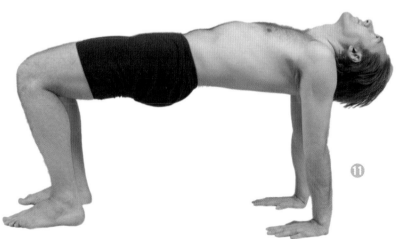

10. If trying to keep your feet on the floor makes your chest feel constricted, do Tabletop pose instead ⑪, with your feet directly under your bent knees and your palms right under your shoulders. Both *Purvottanasana* and Tabletop are excellent platforms for practicing Breath of Fire (p. 74).

Richard Miller

Cow-Face Pose
(Gomukhasana)

Richard Miller insisted on smiling for this photograph. Although in his thirty years as a clinical psychologist and yoga teacher he has studied with the most exacting of asana masters, the best posture to his practiced eye is one that is easy, permissive, and joyous. "When I'm teaching a person a pose," he says, "I'm always asking, 'Is there a sense of delight, wonder, and satisfaction in this moment, or are you hoping to find it in the next moment? How can you adapt the pose so that right now you could die with the face of satisfied desire?'"

Richard's own search for his "face of satisfied desire," a favorite quote of his from the fourteenth-century poet Kabir, began at age thirteen, when he had a sudden sense that he was not separate from anything around him. An abiding yen for that awareness propelled him through multiple fields of study—each of them returning to that same path of inquiry.

In 1970, as a young psychotherapist in training, Richard attended his first yoga class at the Integral Yoga Institute in San Francisco. "I went there hoping to meet people," he says. "But the class was conducted in silence." He floated home anyway, having become newly reacquainted with himself and with the sense of oneness he'd known as a boy.

Richard's propensity for self-inquiry was nurtured by his supervisor, an Asian woman raised on the tenets of Buddhism and yoga. So right from the start, body, mind, and spirituality were being integrated into his studies. "I never felt a disparity between yoga and psychology," Richard says. "Instead, I was interested in how the two came together." They came together with a bang in the form of the mercurial Indian asana master Bikram Choudhury (p. 120), whose tutelage Richard sought out in early 1973.

Bikram, newly arrived in San Francisco, dismissed Richard as a "lazy American" who would not be able to withstand the discipline. "That's just what he does," Richard says with

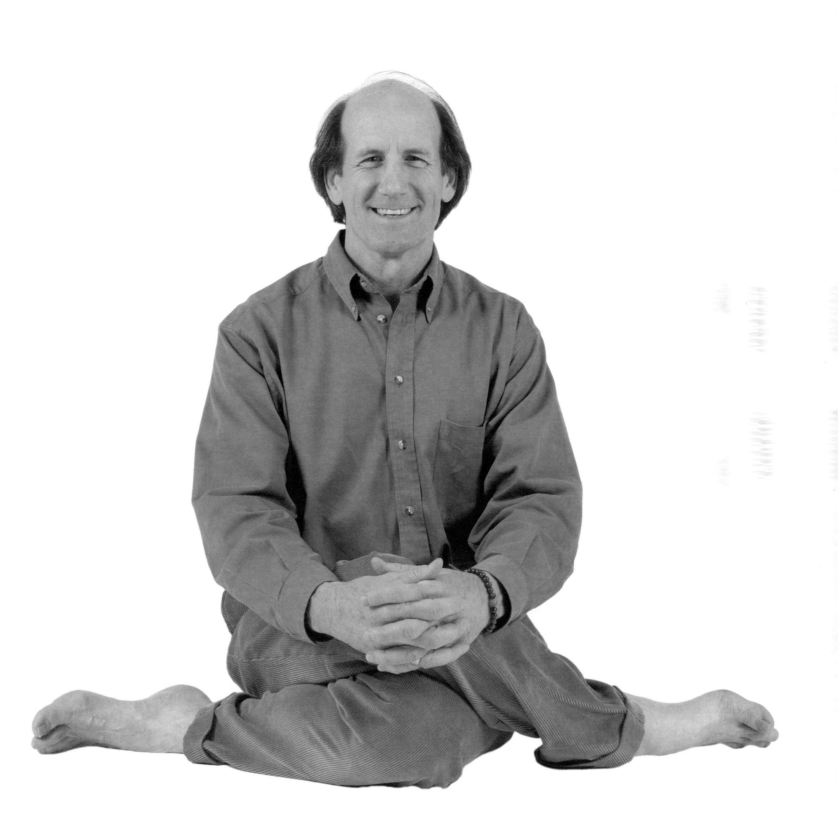

a laugh. "But it was a challenge I felt interested to rise to." Richard found the method highly strengthening physically and mentally, and for a year he studied with Bikram three to four times a week. He even took over teaching his classes when Bikram moved to Los Angeles in 1974. Meanwhile, though, he'd started studying around—with advanced teachers of the Iyengar system, with Swami Bua (an early guru for many Americans in San Francisco and later in New York), and with the Bay Area yoga teacher Joel Kramer.

From 1968 through 1970 Kramer had been the yogi-in-residence at Esalen Institute, the quintessential New Age spiritual retreat center on the cliffs of Big Sur in California. Kramer had forged his own path through reading and Self-study, "but he also had one of those bodies that could wrap itself in any direction," Richard says. "And he had his own style of using breath and energy to open the body and mind. It wasn't 'What are the rules?' but 'What is your actual firsthand experience?' That combined perfectly with my psychology studies."

Kramer also taught Richard to integrate audible *ujjayi* breathing techniques into asana practice, which did not go over well in the Bikram or Iyengar camps. "At Bikram's I was told to stop teaching the breathing or leave. I responded that I couldn't stop breathing, so I'd better leave." And during a long-held Warrior pose at the Iyengar Institute, Richard says, a woman to his left turned to him and hissed," 'What are you doing?' I said, 'I'm breathing.' Nobody around me knew what *ujjayi* was or why anybody would do it."

THE YOGA OF THE POSE: "It feels good. I would say it feels delicious. And I love the opening it brings in my spine and shoulders. To me *Gomukhasana* is one of those poses that feel like dessert. I taught the pose in class once, and I kept saying, 'Find your face of satisified desire,' and one of the students came up afterward and said, 'I don't know about you, honey, but I couldn't find no satisfaction.' Then after class a few weeks later she came up to me and said, 'You know, I found my satisfaction!' In that evening she began to feel her deliciousness."

HOW STUDENTS COMMONLY MISS IT: "When they experience unnecessary discomfort in the pose and cannot inquire as to why that's so. Is it that the body right now isn't able to do *Gomukhasana* in this way—in which case we need to find a variation they can feel comfortable in at this point in time—or is striving in the mind creating the discomfort they're feeling in the body? Look and see if you're causing the pain by striving to be something you're not. It's that constant going inward, your own firsthand experience, that is your teacher."

HOW TO MAKE SURE YOU CONNECT: "Adjust and adapt so you can discover how to be in this moment, in this body, in this disposition, free of fear, free of striving—just open. Back out; make it simpler. Appreciate an advanced *Gomukhasana* variation you may see in a book as a beautiful picture, but come into your own body and sense your own artistic adaptation. In all the teachers I've learned from, what I've seen is there's no right way of doing a pose. So rather than be caught in the thinking mind, open to feeling the body.

"Use the skills of an outer teacher to learn adaptations you might not come to because you're a beginner. Sit on a blanket to get more comfortable or abandon the pose for others that will help you work toward it. Each asana helps open another part of the body to its essence of sensation and aliveness. When the body functions in wholeness, the mind will experience its freedom. Then we can live our non-separate nature moment to moment— which is the true aim of our yoga practice."

In 1974 Richard opened his own yoga center in Marin County. For the next five years he taught yoga, studied acupuncture, saw private psychotherapy clients, wrote articles for the newly founded *Yoga Journal*, and spent as many as five hours a day in hatha yoga practices. "I was able to do extraordinary things physically with asana and with my breath in *pranayama*," he recalls. "But at one point I was holding my leg behind my head and I thought, If I walk out the door after class and get hit by a car and lose all this flexibility, I'm no better for having had it. In that moment I realized that flexibility and strength are passing phenomena, and I was more interested in, Who is this 'I' experiencing it all? How do suffering and separation from that Self arise, and how are they sustained? So while each hatha yoga teaching I received felt like a tremendous gift, none was giving me what I was after."

In 1979 Ian Rawlinson, a British student of the Viniyoga master T.K.V. Desikachar, came to teach at Richard's studio. When Rawlinson left for Madras to study with his teacher, Richard asked if he would take a letter of introduction on his behalf. Two months later Richard was in India.

"When I met Desikachar, there was a sense of coming home," Richard says. "His teachings were tremendously comprehensive." They entailed study of the body, breath, chanting, the *Sutras,* yoga therapy, and a lot of one-to-one tuition." The therapeutic applications of yoga had long interested Richard, so between classes, he would bicycle over to Desikachar's clinic, the Krishnamacharya Yoga Mandiram, and pore over the lessons that had been prescribed for various ailments. "I received an education in using yoga to heal sciatica, back injuries, and all sorts of medical and psychological conditions," he says.

Back in California, Richard was completing work toward becoming a licensed acupuncturist, when he came to understand that his true interest lay in how patients responded psychologically to the treatments. So he went back for a Ph.D. in clin-

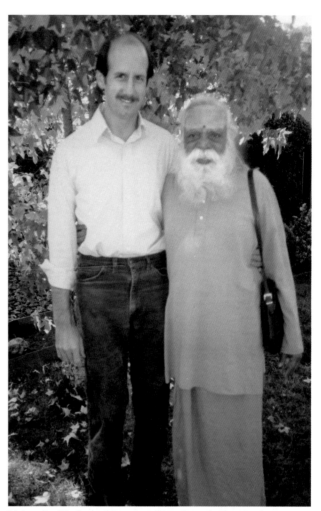

Richard with Swami Bua in Mill Valley, California, in 1984. The Swami, said to be 115 years old, currently lives and teaches seven days a week in New York City.

ical psychology, continuing meanwhile to run his yoga studio and to journey annually to Madras for further study with Desikachar. Then, one autumn evening in 1984, a friend invited Richard to attend a talk by an Austrian named Jean Klein. Klein was a teacher of Advaita, or nondualism, a branch of yoga philosophy predicated on the state of oneness that Richard longed to inhabit. Although Richard was already an avid reader of Advaita texts and philosophy, Klein's talk made him realize that he had found the teacher he'd been searching for all his life.

Klein, who had studied with Desikachar's father, Krishnamacharya, in the early 1950s, integrated hatha yoga, breathing, and meditation "in

Cow-Face Pose *(Gomukhasana)*

Practicing Cow-Face Pose *(Gomukhasana)*

1. From a hands-and-knees position, slip your left knee directly behind your right knee, part the shins, and lower your seat to the floor ❶ or, if that is not possible, onto a block ❷. Keep your knees stacked as best you can and draw your left foot out parallel to your right foot so they emerge equidistant from each thigh. Use calm, deep *ujjayi* breath to sink both hips evenly to the floor.

2. Next do whatever furthers the expansion for you. Stay seated with your eyes closed and continue to breathe deeply. Or walk your hands out in front of you and fold over your legs ❸, leading with your heart. Keep reaching your seat toward the floor as you relax through the shoulders and neck.

3. Like most asanas, *Gomukhasana* works on a variety of muscle groups simultaneously and can challenge you in a variety of ways. If your hips are so tight that you cannot arrange your knees in this position, Richard Miller suggests a reclining Ankle-to-Knee pose ❹ to open the pelvis and hips more gently. Lie on your back, bend your left knee toward your chest, and cross your right ankle above your left knee. Thread your right arm between your legs and your left arm around your left leg, clasping your hands behind your left thigh. Draw your legs toward your chest, resisting the right thigh with the right elbow and keeping the left shin parallel to the floor with the foot flexed. Press your shoulders evenly into the floor.

4. If bowing forward in the pose is difficult because of tightness in the lower back, Richard recommends stretching those muscles in a bent-knee *Uttanasana* ❺ or Child's pose ❻.

a beautiful way that kept the inquiry going no matter what," Richard says. His teachings were really about not-doing, and they possessed a directness and sensibility that penetrated Richard's own practice and teaching immediately and forever.

"The project is to awaken to our true nature," Richard says, "and all these practices—*pranayama*, hatha yoga, yoga therapy, meditation, and even psychotherapy—help support that. When an emotion, memory, or psychological issue arises in the body during asana, we can learn to meet it at the level of pure sensation. If we just meet it as it is and welcome it, rather than try to push it away or get involved in analyzing it, we will see that its inherent nature is change, and it will blossom and dissolve. We can say, 'I'm afraid,' or we can say, 'Fear is arising; can I be with this?' So we use the posture to invite feelings we might otherwise have only in situations where we're not prepared."

One of Richard's clients is still dealing with terror stemming from the 9/11 disaster. "During *Virabhadrasana* or Handstand, we let fear in as her ally, as a messenger, rather than just something we're trying to get rid of. So the fear she now feels when she gets on a plane helps bring her back to that moment she hasn't completely digested. Her fear has actually become her friend."

Many American yoga practitioners today give short shrift to such deeper inquiry, and that's fine with Richard. "They're in their first steps, and if they ultimately start to feel that something is missing in their practice, they'll look around and see the next step and the next. So it's all perfect, a wonderful paradox. Awareness is not something we develop. It's something we all are and fall into. And because we're not separate, we're all already home. So everyone will come home—whether it's on their deathbed or at some other time. It's a done deal."

As is true for every teacher, what Richard shares is a patchwork of his experiences. Asana, meditation, breath work, yoga therapy, psychotherapy, teaching, practice, marriage, and fatherhood—it all melds into his understanding and transmission of yoga in an increasingly seamless way. You could say there is no separation.

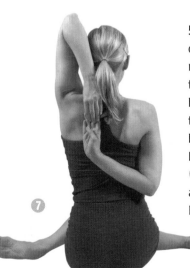

5. *Gomukhasana* classically includes the shoulder-opener shown at left ❼. If your right knee is on top, reach your left arm straight up to the ceiling and bend the elbow, bringing the palm between the shoulder blades. Take your right hand to your left elbow to work the hand down lower. Then swim your right arm back behind you and reach up to take the left fingers or wrist. If clasping the hands is not possible, use a strap or towel ❽. Draw the shoulders away from the ears and open across the chest as you sit tall or fold forward over your legs.

Sharon Gannon

One-legged King Pigeon
(Eka Pada Rajakapotasana variation)

A decade before she discovered yoga's physical practices, Sharon Gannon found herself drawn deeply to its literature. The heat of that passion continues to fuel every class she teaches at Jivamukti Yoga Center in New York City, the school she cofounded in 1989 with her partner, David Life. There and in workshops as far afield as Japan, Gannon mixes pop and sacred music with readings from scriptures to ensure that the practice becomes more than physical for everyone in the room. "The body is a way to reach into the interior of the mind and move toward the source," she says.

Sharon began studying Sanskrit texts and practicing meditation in 1973 when she was a dance student at the University of Washington. For her the studies were absolutely complementary. "I came to dance and to contemplative practice for the same reason: because I was interested in prying beneath the surface of the reality we experience every day," she says. "Through the readings and chanting, I was investigating, among other things, what makes form form. Dance was the most challenging way I could find at the time to experiment with the outer form as a reflection of what is going on inside. Your resistances, feelings of incompetence, jealousy, sadness, your competitive nature—all that flies up in your face in a rigorous university dance program. And that, as I came to find, is what happens in a good yoga class."

Her first experience with hatha yoga, a class she took on a visit to Santa Cruz, California, in 1972, did not hint at that level of intensity. "The class was one of those rolling-around-on-the-floor-feeling-good kind of things," she says. "You know, twisting here, twisting there, candles in the room. We chanted Om and they served hot milk with turmeric afterward. I liked it. It was nice. But nobody told me anything about what was going on. And dance was a lot more challenging physically, emotionally, and spiritually."

During and after college, Sharon's performances as a dancer, violinist, and vocalist melded traditions in the same way her yoga teaching eventually would. The guiding prin-

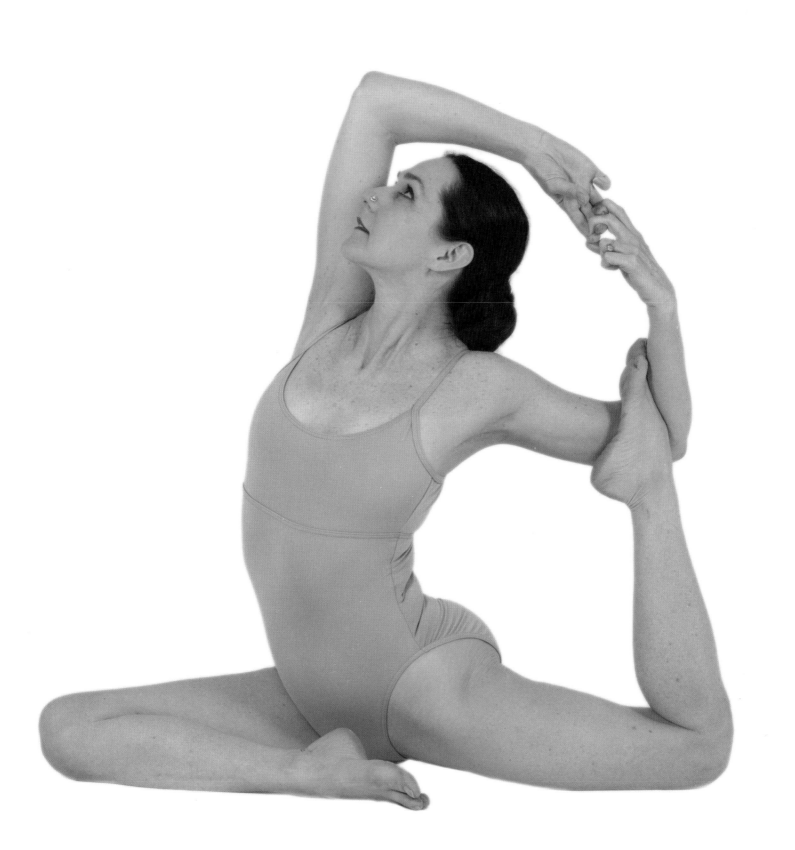

ciple was even the same: to raise consciousness, she says. "My art continued to draw on the things I had been studying all along, including Vedantic teachings and chanting. But I had become disillusioned with what art had become—just another commodity. It bothered me to be onstage and have people sit in the audience just watching or criticizing. I wanted to give them the tools to have the experience themselves."

The toolbox was prized open when she moved to New York City in 1983. After she and her band performed at a café owned by David Life, Sharon wound up waitressing there while continuing to dance, play music, and record. During that time, she was in great pain from a back injury that

wouldn't quit, despite repeated visits to a host of physicians. The last, an orthopedic surgeon, strongly recommended an operation.

Sharon considered having the surgery and talked it over with a fellow waitress at the café, named Tara Rose. Tara happened to be a yoga teacher and suggested that Sharon come to class. "I just laughed and said, 'I don't think so; I can hardly stand up!'" Sharon says. But when she finally gave it a try, the experience thrilled her on a variety of levels—not least because of how it eased her discomfort. "I went back and told the surgeon, and he said, 'You know, if you're getting some relief, why don't you go with the yoga? Because I can't guarantee that after the surgery

THE YOGA OF THE POSE: "I love the feeling of begin grounded through the terrestrial force of gravity and how that connection enables me to tap into the celestial force by lifting my heart and emotions to that which is eternally joyful."

HOW STUDENTS COMMONLY MISS IT: *"Eka Pada Rajakapotasana* is a backbend, but in order to bend back in this pose, you must first of all have a solid and good connection to the earth. And for that, you have to have your hips open.

"So the biggest way people miss the pose is by being extremely tight in the hips. And if you can't sit still long enough to work on opening the hips, you're not going to be able to move out of your limited range of motion toward service to others—which is the metaphor of backbending: to come out of yourself.

"What inhibits people from working on their hips is thinking it's not important in the bigger scheme of things. Opening the hips is useful if you want to be able to sit with some sense of ease and comfort, which is only important to someone who wants to gain the necessary calmness to serve the earth, humanity, and God. Not everybody wants that."

HOW TO MAKE SURE YOU CONNECT: "Show up—that's the practice. Do this regularly, and you will change, you will gain flexibility. There's no prerequisite other than that. You have a sincere desire to change, so you come and you do the practice. Just sitting and breathing long and often enough in Pigeon preparation—staying there even two or three breaths is a good start—will gradually open the hips.

"To begin to release the psoas is to begin to step forward with grace and fearlessness into your own future. The psoas is connected to your fight-or-flight reflex. It's helpful to address that area of the body, because it connects us to something deeper and more profound on a psychological level. Hip openers, like all the asanas, release tremendous energy on a physical level that has an effect on your consciousness because consciousness is chemical. By practicing them, you gain control over your own state of mind. So it's not just making you feel better in your body; it's giving you more clarity about your present condition, a more expansive view. Any psychologist will tell you that if you can expand your perception of your condition, you will feel better. That's what Pigeon can teach you to do."

Practicing Pigeon
(Eka Pada Rajakapotasana)

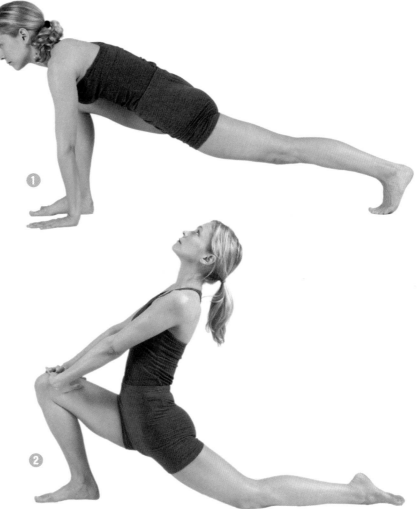

1. Pigeon is a double whammy of a hip opener in that it simultaneously works to release tightness in the muscles in the back and side of your front hip and in the front of your back hip and thigh. The process begins when you step into lunge pose during Sun Salutations ❶ and intensifies when you send the hips and pelvis forward and down in Knee-down Lunge ❷.

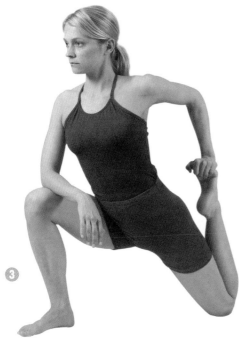

2. Pressing the left foot toward the left buttock from Knee-down Lunge ❸ approximates the deep stretch of the iliopsoas muscle Sharon Gannon is demonstrating. Because we sit so much in chairs and engage in exercise programs that emphasize repetitive hip flexion—such as running or the use of step machines—Americans tend to have shortened iliopsoas muscles, which skews alignment in the spine and hip joints. Yoga comprises the counteractions of stretching and strengthening—here of the intricate muscles around the hips, pelvis, and sacrum—so that the body remains a healthy vessel for the spirit within.

One-legged King Pigeon *(Eka Pada Rajakapotasana* variation*)*

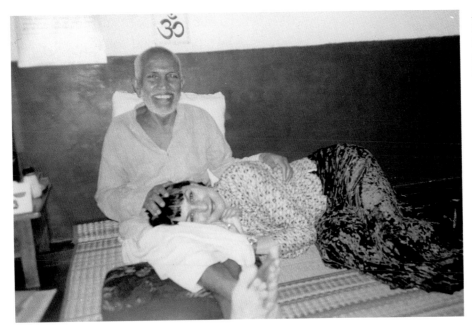

"Spoken word, lyrics, and readings are very important in classes," she says. "I have always believed that the language we use has an impact on the reality we live. And since I'm only one person having one experience of reality, I like to draw from other people and other artists."

you'll even have the flexibility you have now.'" After two years of steady and careful practice, Sharon built up the muscles in her back until they held the bones in place. The experience gave her extra motivation to seek out and spread the good word.

For the next two years Sharon took yoga classes all over the city in an effort to find the richly textured experience she envisioned. "Intuitively Tara was fantastic," she says, "but she didn't know about the history, philosophy, and chanting I had been interested in, which really began to fall together once I started the physical practice." Even the Sivananda-style practice, which Sharon became certified to teach in 1986 and which places heavy emphasis on the study and relevance of scriptures, maintained strict separation between those aspects and asana. Sharon sought the expression of their simultaneity.

"I had had some amazing mystical experiences while doing hatha yoga, so it didn't make sense to me that there was no direction in that regard given in the class," she says. "It seemed incorrect that I had to do it on my own outside of class." So from the time she began teaching in 1987, Sharon made certain that the words she spoke were both instructional and inspirational.

The artists Sharon selects can be surprising. In a class she taught one Valentine's Day, the overly dramatic voice of the '50s pop tenor Mario Lanza brought laughter to students doing an extremely unfunny posture sequence that had the whole class sweating bullets. "But it did the trick," Sharon notes. "I enjoy taking things out of their original context and seeing if they can be molded into something useful for a higher experience or a deeper delve."

For all her pop-culture references, Sharon's teachings unequivocally rely on the texts that called to her three decades ago. "Yoga is five thousand years old, but remember, it's been going *on* for five thousand years. It's a living tradition. It's something you do that helps you in life, something that promotes a direction that is positive and toward the source—which some people call God.

"For the most part it is very difficult for people to devote efforts to God. Who is God? Where does He live? What does He look like? But there are other devotions: world peace, nonharming, ridding yourself of anger and self-centeredness— these kinds of goals are a good starting point. Then your perception becomes more clear about difficult issues like God and the world."

One major reason Sharon chose to become a yoga teacher was to promulgate the practice of *ahimsa,* or nonharming, in a proactive way. "Yogis have always striven to live in harmony with the environment," she says. "From the beginning, their role in society has been as a protector and devotee of Mother Earth." Yoga originated with Lord Shiva, she points out, who is also called Pashupati, the protector of animals. Sharon has seen to it that Jivamukti teachings stress concern for the environment, vegetarianism, and political activism as essential aspects of the practice.

The approach has created controversy. "When we presented these issues at yoga conferences, other participants warned me that I could alienate potential students," Sharon says. But that didn't stop her. In 1999 she founded Animal Mukti, New York City's first free spay and neuter clinic, which has reduced by thirty percent the number of dogs and cats euthanized in the city each year. She also brought the politics of yoga to her music. In 2003 she released a CD that mixes original music from

3. To move into Pigeon preparation, place your right knee between your palms and your right heel toward the front of your left hip ④. The often heard instruction to lay the shin parallel to the front edge of the mat may not be possible for you, but you can explore the concept by using props ⑤. Make certain your right foot is not under your thigh, but aiming out to the left, with the right thigh roughly parallel to the right edge of your mat. Some teachers recommend taking your right knee a little out to right so it is under your right shoulder, as pictured left ④. Try it both ways to glean the wisdom of each instruction.

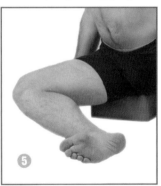

4. Ultimately the back of your right thigh and the front of your left thigh should rest comfortably on the floor. To learn how that feels, place a block or a blanket under your right buttock ⑥ and begin to release forward evenly over your thigh. Forward bending in Pigeon preparation initiates a deep stretch of the lateral hip muscles that can inhibit the outward rotation necessary to "connect with the earth," which Sharon says is key in the pose. Send *prana,* life-force energy, in the form of calm, regulated breath, into areas of constriction.

the band that brought her to New York with lecture excerpts from activists such as John Robbins (p. 176), whose work promoting vegetarianism, animal rights, and sustainable agriculture matches Sharon's definition of yoga.

What Sharon wants is to wake people up. Her asana classes are hard on purpose—"Bend your knee like you *mean* to do it!" she scolds halfhearted warriors—but her aim is sweet and true. "When yoga practices become dry, they're never going to work; they are not going to make you ultimately happy," she says. "So we try to level the situation every now and then in class. The source of the

universe is bliss; this is what it says in the Taittiriya Upanishad. And if you want to realize that, there must be something of it in your daily life, even if it's just a glimmer."

So the Jivamukti prescription is to get heavy into yoga and lighten up as you do. "Since we all fall victim to taking ourselves too seriously—myself included—that's the first thing to watch out for," Sharon says. "Whenever you feel that creeping in, pull the rug out from underneath yourself. Stand on your head. Go see a Marx Brothers movie." (Or listen to Mario Lanza while sweating bullets of purification on Valentine's Day.)

5. In order not to collapse into the right buttock ❼, flex your left toes under and press strongly through the back heel till the knee and thigh are lifted ❽. Use your straight leg as a lever to drop both hips evenly toward the floor and bow forward this way for a few breaths in order to ensure correct alignment. Continue to roll the inner left thigh up toward the ceiling as you ease your outer right hip and buttock toward the floor. Lengthen from the navel to the sternum, and from the navel to the back big toe.

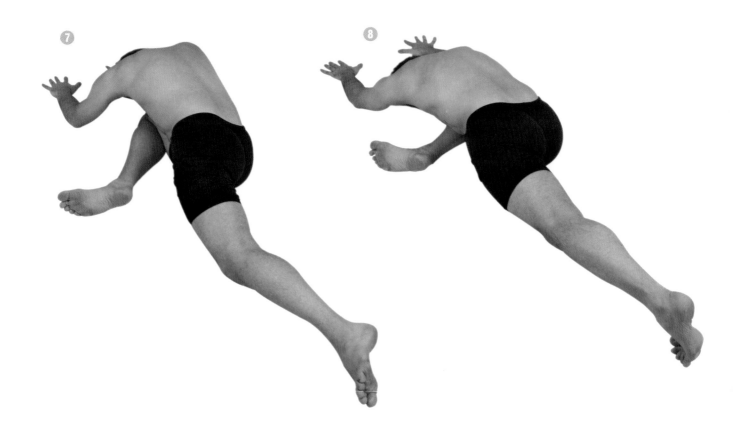

Sharon applauds the growing popularity of yoga in America. "I really believe it is a part of our culture now because it is much needed," she says. "But if there isn't an element of devotion, of offering your efforts to some higher force than your own personal motivation, then the practice can fall flat and even have negative consequences." One way to avoid that snare, she says, is to look to the "saints and sages who have brought light into human consciousness"—which is why she and David named their school after the Sanskrit term *jivan-mukti,* "liberated being."

These sages and saints smile down at you from the altar as you practice in Jivamukti's main classroom. "We want to turn people on to the teachers we have had and are inspired by daily," Sharon says. The ever expanding iconography—which includes the Astanga Yoga patriarch Pattabhi Jois, T. Krishnamacharya, Bob Dylan, Sri Brahmananda Sarasvati, and Ram Dass—forms a chronicle of American yoga that is at once personal and collective. It is also a testament to the vibrant expression of the discipline that Sharon Gannon longed to hear and finally made.

6. When you sit up once again, take your fingertips back by your hips and puff your chest forward of your shoulders like a bird ⑨. This easy stretch across the front of the chest and shoulders allows you to begin to move into the deep backbend that Sharon says defines this pose. "In the full *Eka Pada Rajakapotasana* ⑩ the foot has to make contact with the head." Shoulder-openers like *Gomukhasana* (p. 143) and *Dhanurasana* (p. 127) move us gradually toward such openness.

Gary Kraftsow
Headstand
(Sirsasana)

In a workshop at a large yoga conference in the States, Gary Kraftsow asked participants to choose Sanskrit or English for the chanted portion of his teachings. When the show of hands was noncommittal, the longtime student of Vedic texts weighed in with his own preference. He'd opt for English. "Yoga is really nonsectarian," he says, "and it may not be appropriate to ask a devout Christian to do Hindu chants. The ability to help a person of deep Catholic or Jewish faith—or someone who is an atheist—to make a spiritual connection increases tremendously if you adapt the practices to that person."

Adapting the practice to the person is the essence of Viniyoga, the methodology Gary found his way to three decades ago. As a nineteen-year-old religious studies student at Colgate University, Gary took a yoga class to fulfill a physical education requirement. Within six months he had headed off to India in search of his teacher's teacher: T. Krishnamacharya (p. 45).

It was Krishnamacharya's son T.K.V. Desikachar who began training the young Kraftsow to carry on his father's tradition, which stresses selected application of asana, *pranayama,* meditation, yoga therapy, and spiritual practice for particular people in particular phases of life. Although group classes comprise much of Gary's instruction today, the teacher-training programs he coordinates through his American Viniyoga Institute in Maui, Hawaii, are aimed at individualized *cikitsa* or yoga therapy. Postures are just one aspect of the work.

"Many Western practitioners misunderstand the purpose of asana by taking it out of its original context—which is part of an overall process of transformation at every level—and by making it about performance, measuring progress by how many asanas they can do. Asana is fundamentally about moving awareness in the body and then about moving energy in the body through awareness. So we do asana from the point of view of health. But then we do inner work to deepen our self-understanding through reflection so that we don't keep making the same mistakes over and over again, hurting people—all of that."

It has been said that yoga is not a religion, but the science of religion, an examination that for Gary began in the backyard of his childhood home in Philadelphia. He recalls sitting out under the stars and engaging in an unwitting meditation on nothingness, progressively "disappearing things" in his mind to see what remained. That brand of investigation deepened with age. Gary's master's thesis was on religion and health. "Now with

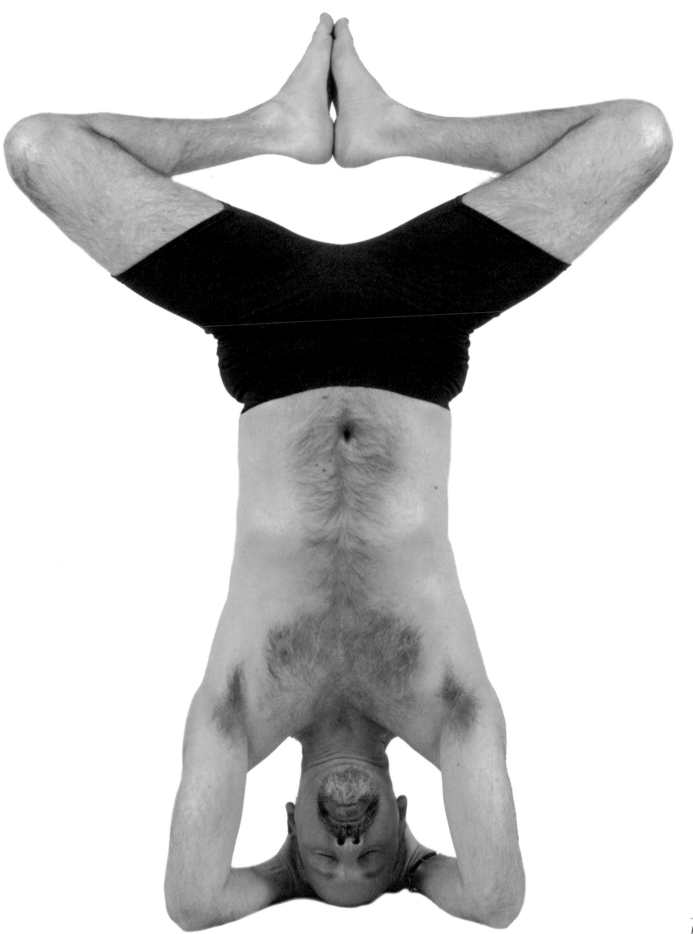

the work Deepak Chopra has done, the connection is obvious, but then people wondered, What is this?" Gary is currently completing a Ph.D. in religious studies. Yet his purview of the implementation of yoga in America is far from academic.

"Part of my dharma, if I have a dharma with regard to yoga, is to train teachers who can convey yoga's power to create not just structural but physiological and psycho-emotional fitness," he says. "Few resources exist in this country to help people understand how they can use the breath to work with physiological problems and balance the emotional state or how meditation and prayer can deepen self-understanding and clarity about their direction for the future."

At the Krishnamacharya Yoga Mandiram in Chennai, India, where Gary has continued to apprentice annually with Desikachar, one-on-one yoga therapy is used to treat people with disorders ranging from depression to heart disease. "It's not an asana gym—it's a clinic recognized by the Ministry of Health," Gary says. "And the clinic trains hospital staff to work with retarded children and effects all kinds of social action." Gary is encouraged by the beginnings of such work in this country. In 2003 he was asked to design protocol for a study on low back pain underwritten by the National Institutes of Health and for another that Harvard Medical School is conducting on chronic anxiety. "And I'm just one person," he says. "There's a lot of work going on in therapy that I think will benefit our society."

Gary has equally high expectations for yoga's ability to redress what he sees as our nation's "crisis of faith." He notes that "few Americans take nourishment from their ancestral heritage. The images, forms, beliefs that gave strength to our

---

THE YOGA OF THE POSE: "The effect of *viparita karani*, or active reversal, is said to tone the vital organs, stimulate the endocrine glands, and promote balanced and effective function of our entire physiology. Headstand is considered the king of the postures; it's very powerful. It strengthens your spinal and respiratory musculature, and it has been shown to regulate blood pressure. On a subjective level people experience calmness, focus, and centeredness after headstand. So if you can do it safely, it's a wonderful posture."

HOW STUDENTS COMMONLY MISS IT: "By going into the pose when they're not ready—because they're not strong enough in the upper back or neck, they're overweight in their hips, their low back is excessively bowed, or the upper back is excessively rounded. To stay up for a length of time without stress to the structure requires a fairly well-developed body. You must be able to bring the natural curves of the spine into maximum vertical alignment relative to the base of the posture—in this case the top of the head, the forearms, and the hands."

HOW TO MAKE SURE YOU CONNECT: "To use Headstand safely, people have to understand how to prepare and compensate for the pose and how to assess their body to know if it's a posture that's appropriate for them to explore. The most common injuries in asana practice are to the joints—in the case of Headstand, the intervertebral joints in the neck. Since long, incorrect practice of Headstand can lead to cervical disc degeneration, in my view the way to know if you're ready for it is when the teacher tells you.

"But in general: Move slowly and don't be driven by an external image of the pose that you cannot comfortably attain. If you always use the wall to come up, you can suffer posterior cervical injury. If you always kick up, you won't necessarily gain the control required to stay in the posture safely. Ideally when you're in Headstand, you are not efforting; you should be able to come into a place where you go into a deep meditative state with long breathing."

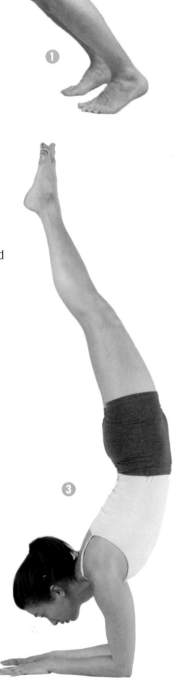

Practicing Headstand *(Sirsasana)*

1. To avoid injuring the neck in Headstand, it is necessary to strengthen the trapezius, biceps, and forearm muscles, which should bear much more weight than the head—especially as we learn the pose. Downward-Facing Dog **1**, Handstand **2**, and the setup for Forearm Stand **3** strengthen these muscles and train you to make space between the shoulders and ears, an essential aspect of *Sirsasana*.

families two, three, four, five generations back, do not work for most of us anymore. The yoga tradition has evolved profound tools to help people find true sources within ourselves without having to join a club of orthodoxy or make a partial or really sort of false jump into becoming a Hindu or a Buddhist."

The tools Gary refers to are the core teachings of the *Yoga Sutras* of Patanjali (p. 56), which he believes must be explored experientially and evenhandedly in order to be effective. "I don't want to say asana practice can't take you to God,

but what's taking you to God isn't the asanas. It's you and your intention and your heart connection. Cultivating that is not simply through refining the physical details of your asana practice."

The science of yoga—specifically the observances of *tapas* (purification arising from disciplined practice), *svadhyaya* (Self-discovery through reflection and study), and *Isvara pranidhana* (dedication to the highest)—aims to alleviate the causes of suffering that stem from incorrect perception. The Self-study Patanjali specified involved the recitation of scripture, a calming, expansive practice

2. One Headstand preparation Gary recommends is a *Parivrtta Trikonasana* variation that ascertains the necessary mobility and readiness in the upper spine and neck. Stand with your feet spread wider than your shoulders and with your arms out to the sides and parallel to the floor ❹. As you exhale, bend forward and twist to the right, bringing the left hand to the floor and the right arm up to the ceiling. Look down at the left hand ❺.

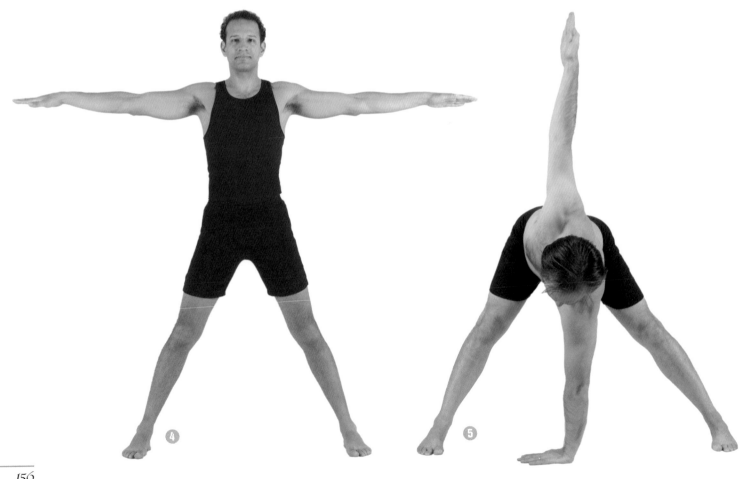

In the following excerpt Sylvia Hellman, an early Western disciple of Swami Sivananda in the 1940s, asks her guru why asana practice—and Headstand in particular—is important to spiritual growth.

"Imagine that you are standing on your head," Swami Sivananda said to me. "What can you observe?"

In my imagination I put myself in that position and I said, "Well, everything is upside down."

"Very good, very good," Master said. "And what is upside down? Tell me all about it."

"Well, my immediate surroundings, everything that is within the vision of my eye, and that is as far as I can observe."

Master said, "How does that apply in life?"

I didn't know what he was talking about, so he had to help me by saying,"People have opposed you, haven't they?"

"Oh, yes, plenty."

"They believe the opposite to what you believe. Well, the headstand can help you by making you your own opponent. You take your cherished beliefs, go right in the opposite direction, just as you would oppose another person. If you can do this, the result will be a greater accuracy of what you believe to be true, a better balance. You will not be flustered, you will not be angered if anybody opposes you. You will also not be so foolish as to say that you have all the answers."

—Swami Sivananda Radha *Radha: Diary of a Woman's Search*

3. On an inhale look up at your right hand ⑥. Then exhale and take the right arm over your ear, gazing into the palm ⑦. As you inhale, stretch the arm back up to the ceiling ⑥, then exhale and look back down at your left hand ⑤. Inhale up to stand ④, and repeat on the other side. Move dynamically through this series six times per side alternately.

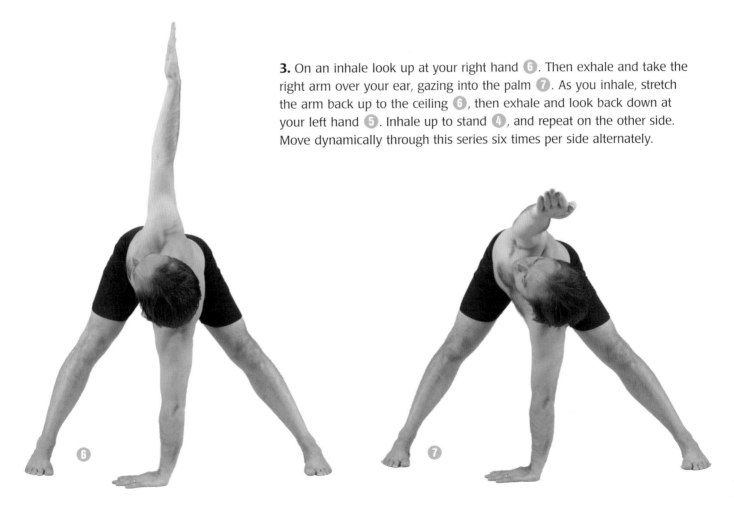

⑥   ⑦

Headstand *(Sirsasana)*

that has the same effects today as it did five millennia ago. That's why Gary incorporates chanting into his teachings in a way everybody can connect with.

"Since I'm American, not Indian, what I'm going to teach will be influenced by that base in culture," he says. "The Indian approach is a guru-disciple, teacher-student, master-servant, Brahmin-non-Brahmin modality. Ours is egalitarian; it's a very different way of relating and appreciating material. For us it's information we can apply in our lives in an effective way."

The words that Gary chanted during his workshop were love, trust, freedom, harmony, abundance, health, peace, security, fun, joy, gratitude, and contentment. If they sound far less New Agey in Sanskrit, they have a powerful reverberation in English when combined with breathing and visualization techniques tempered by gentle asana. But in any language the sentiment of the twelve words Gary chose is as ancient as mankind. And since they form the wish list of all beings everywhere, Gary does what he can to drive that awareness home.

4. A Headstand preparation from the Sivananda tradition is Dolphin. Begin by hugging your elbows under the shoulders ❽, then extend your forearms, and make one fist with both hands. Straighten your legs behind you until your body is parallel to the floor. On an inhale move your heart and chin forward of your thumbs ❾. As you exhale, press your hips up and back ❿. Repeat as many times as you can in order to build strength for Headstand. Remember: Keep the chest open, not collapsed, and let the chest move the shoulders forward, instead of vice versa.

WHEN NOT TO INVERT

Inversions are key to a well-rounded yoga practice—but they may not always be appropriate for you. "If an inversion causes pain, that's a contraindication to doing it," says Gail Dubinsky, M.D., a physician and yoga teacher in Sebastopol, California. "Either you figure out why it's hurting and make it stop, or you don't do it. That's number one, no matter what your condition or diagnosis is."

A specialist in osteopathic medicine, Dr. Dubinsky found out that the ten- and fifteen-minute Headstands required in the teacher training program she was enrolled in were doing her damage. She had been ignoring the lingering tension she experienced for about an hour after Headstand and was surprised when an examination by a physical therapist determined she had a severely degenerated cervical disk, resulting in a pinched nerve.

"The main caveat in inversions is they should be done by prepared practitioners who have the necessary strength and opening in their upper back, shoulder girdle, and chest. If you have any suspicion of a cervical spine condition that could be adversely impacted by Headstand or Shoulder Stand, you should be examined by a health practitioner specializing in orthopedic conditions."

Other red flags may include any type of compressed or herniated disks, glaucoma, and hypertension—although people whose mild to moderate high blood pressure is controlled by medication can be introduced slowly to gentle inversions like *Viparita Karani*, Dr. Dubinsky says. When it comes to Shoulder Stand, you can always modify, she says, but she believes that Headstand is never advisable for people with facet problems, where the compression is bone-on-bone. And while inversions like Handstand and Forearm Stand are fine for practitioners who should not bear weight on the head, they can be more dangerous than Headstand for glaucoma patients. So at-risk practitioners should approach inversions under the supervision of a knowledgeable yoga teacher, Dr. Dubinsky says.

In the minds of many yoga teachers and practitioners, a definite contraindication to turning upside down is menstruation. When you are in the "moon club," as Judith Lasater calls it, "do forward bends and quiet poses and not strenuous backbends and standing poses. Because I'm a bit of a rebel, I used to do active poses and inversions anyway, and my period would stop, or become too heavy. We tell everybody yoga works, but then we act like it doesn't! These poses really have an effect, and to pretend we're the same as men is to ignore the reality of female physiology." There is a blood vessel within the ligament that holds the uterus in place that gets stretched and occluded when you turn upside down, Judith points out. "So when you turn back right side up, it backs up and floods."

Although Beryl Bender Birch says a vigorous practice kept her cycle regular and her hormone levels well balanced, she agrees that inversions during menstruation are to be avoided. "*Apana* [the downward flow of energy in yoga and *aryuveda*] is doing its work," she says. "It's moving the unfertilized egg out of the body, and you don't want to interrupt that. But my feeling is that to take five breaths in Shoulder Stand or five breaths in Headstand is fine. It always made my reproductive organs feel energized."

While on their cycle, most female yoga practitioners have at one time or another gone ahead and turned upside down in a group asana class. "For women who have issues about menstruation, doing a restorative pose while everyone else is in Shoulder Stand puts this little scarlet M on you," Dr. Dubinsky points out. But ultimately, the women in this book recommend putting the ego and the inversions on hold. "There are so many wonderful poses available: beautiful forward bends, twists, poses that are actually more meditative in nature anyway," Patricia Sullivan says. "And if yoga is to teach us that what we are is beyond the physical, what's the attachment to whether you turn upside down twenty-four days a month as opposed to twenty-eight days? It really comes down to just let it go."

Headstand *(Sirsasana)*

"The end point of yoga—the state of mind in which the perception of the observed is less and less mediated by the conditioning of the observer—is very nonmystical," he says. "It is something everybody has the capacity to experience as the mind becomes less distracted and more refined and purified. It's a matter of coming back to yourself, arriving in your own true nature, discovering who you are, and being interested in that process. As we go deeper into this work, we have a greater ability to understand the dynamics of our relationships and our own strategies of avoidance and denial."

For all his learnedness and immersion in Indic thought, history, literature, and methodology, Gary may be the most American of yoga teachers. He teaches yoga classes in street clothes, which is what he showed up in to be photographed for this book. But in order to clearly demonstrate Headstand he donned a pair of borrowed shorts—not minding a bit that they were something he would not ordinarily wear. "Yoga is the technology of reducing self-importance and opening your heart to something bigger," he notes. In this case, as is often the case with Gary, what was bigger was what he could share.

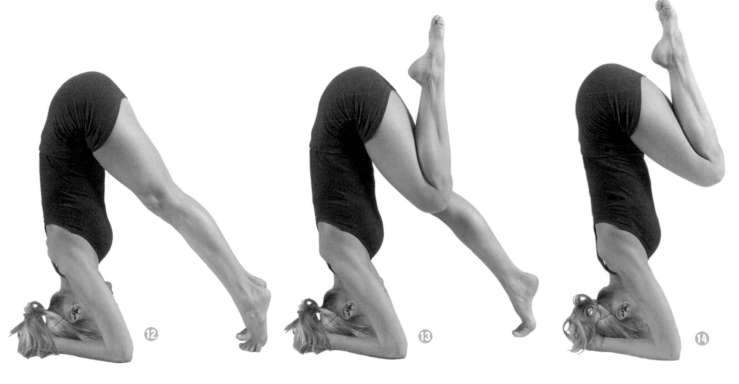

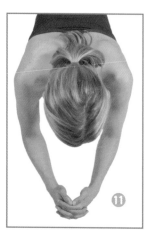

5. Once your Dolphin can swim, try Headstand Preparation. From a kneeling position, hug your elbows on the floor under your shoulders and maintain that width as you extend the forearms and interlace the fingers into a basket, tucking in the bottom pinky ⑪. Keep the roots of the fingers interlocked but separate the palms and place the crown of your head on the floor and the back of your head lightly against the heels of the hands. Press evenly into the outer edges of the wrists and forearms as you lift your hips and slowly tiptoe your feet toward your face, aligning your hips over your shoulders ⑫. See if you can lift your head off the floor here, then lower it back down, maintaining the participation of your forearms and upper arms. Once you feel secure in Headstand Preparation, draw one knee toward your chest ⑬, and then the other ⑭. This is a fine place to work.

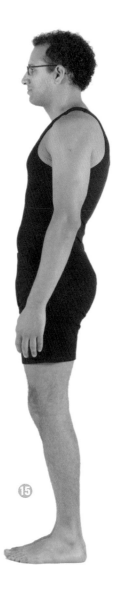

6. Like most things in life, full Headstand is difficult at the start. The first time you go up into the balance will likely be frightening, and staying up will entail herculean effort and a good deal of sweat. But it should never hurt your neck. If it does, come down and keep developing the muscles and alignment you need to do the pose safely. The postural imbalances reflected in how you stand on your feet are exaggerated in Headstand. For someone with an excessively curved thoracic spine 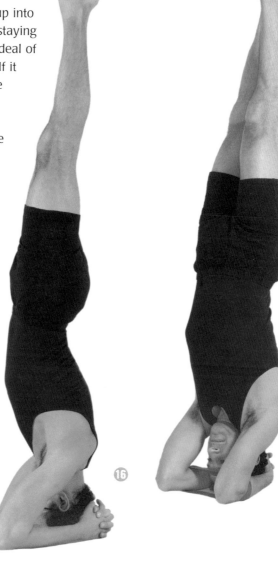, Headstand is inadvisable until the position of the head and neck is improved through the practice of general and specific asanas. One such exercise is the Headless Headstand, in which the strapped elbows redirect pressure from the upper spine into the forearms and shoulder girdle. Working at the wall, follow instructions for Headstand preparation but keep your head lifted off the floor and draw your navel toward your spine to aid the natural *uddiyana bandha* the pose encourages. Then take one foot away from the wall and align your body from the top of your head through your spine to your heel.

7. After Headstand, rest in Child's pose by dropping your seat on your heels and your forehead on the floor. Breathe fully into the back body. If your head doesn't reach the floor, make a pillow with your hands, and if a knee injury makes this restful pose uncomfortable, place padding between the backs of the legs and the buttocks. Shoulder Stand (p. 165) and Half-Wheel are the classic counterposes for Headstand.

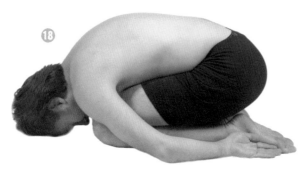

Patricia Sullivan

Plow/Shoulder Stand
(Halasana/
Salamba Sarvangasana)

Patricia Sullivan was teaching yoga asanas—and teaching others how to teach them—for the better part of two decades before she discovered her own calm, steady seat. It was 1976 when she first became fascinated with the precise methodology of B.K.S. Iyengar after watching the asana master give a demonstration in San Francisco's Tilden Park. Over the next decade she made three pilgrimages to Pune to study with him and his daughter Geeta, maturing as a senior instructor at the San Francisco Iyengar Yoga Institute in the process. And although she remains grateful for the lessons of what she acknowledges as a "brilliant method," Patricia ultimately freed herself from its strictures to embrace a style of practice as organic and variegated as the garden that surrounds her Marin County, California, studio.

"It seemed clear to me at some point that I wanted to be able to connect with students in a way that wasn't through stiffness, sternness, intimidation, perfection—that there are other ways to encourage people to seek their depths," Patricia says. That sensibility has surely been heightened by her connection with the Zen priest Edward Espe Brown, her partner since 1984. But she was headed that way regardless.

As the daughter of a naval officer, Patricia spent her high school years in Hawaii, where

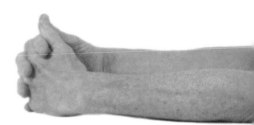

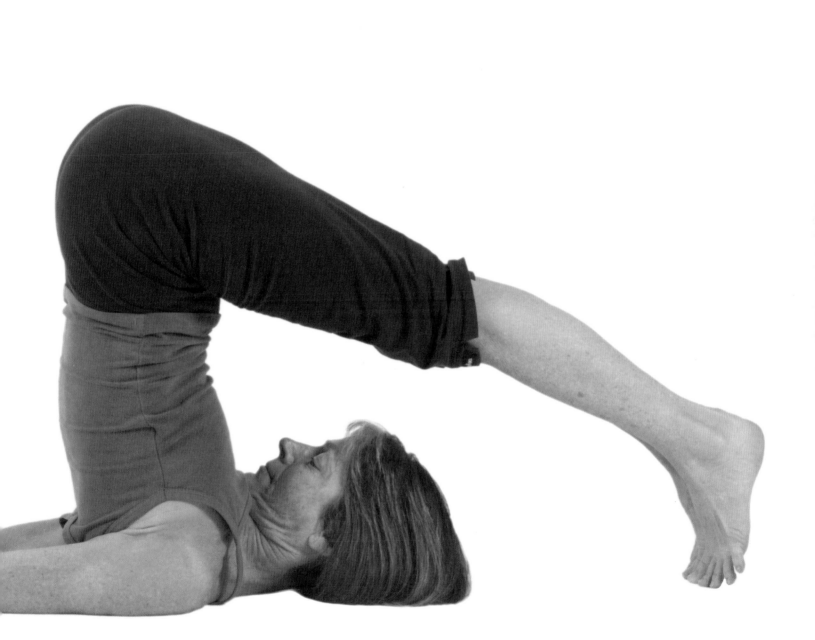

Plow/Shoulder Stand (Halasana/Salamba Sarvangasana)

THE YOGA OF THE POSE: "The wonderful things about Plow are that it's good as a preparation for Shoulder Stand, it's powerful on its own as a pose and for working out high blood pressure situations, and it's also an excellent way to end the *Salamba Sarvangasana* sequence.

"Shoulder Stand is considered the queen of all asanas—*Salamba* means supported and *sarvanga* means all the limbs—because it supports the entire body and flushes all of your systems. It completely reverses the pressure on the digestive organs, and it decreases blood flow to the legs. That's the cleansing aspect of it. But it also increases blood flow into the endocrine glands, so in that sense it's very holistic. And in some sense it embodies what I want yoga to be for people who practice it: It offers something for all aspects of their being."

HOW STUDENTS COMMONLY MISS IT: "For most people it takes a certain amount of time to become comfortable enough in Shoulder Stand so that it's no longer a struggle. It's hard to notice all the benefits if you're just struggling to be there. Many people have a tight neck, and then they are asked to flex it 90 degrees, with peer pressure on top of that to stay up as long as everybody else. Still, I have had a lot of people say, 'I don't like this pose when I'm in it, but I feel good when I come out of it.' Afterward they notice its calming and rejuvenating effect.

"Some students need to work with props but only realize it in hindsight. Even though I was using props and thought I was doing the pose just fine in the early years, I ended up with a lot of neck problems. It took me years to back off on the way I was taught to do it and to search for a way I could do it so that it worked for me."

HOW TO MAKE SURE YOU CONNECT: "Don't compete or try to force the pose. Learn to prepare for it more carefully with long holds of supported Bridge pose, rocking and rolling on the back to soften the back muscles, positions like Cobra that stretch and release the neck, and shoulder openers like *Gomukhasana*. Doing Plow with the feet propped as necessary can enable you to enter Shoulder Stand without being in so much struggle. This can be true even for beginning-level students.

"I'm not an advocate of everybody using props, but I am an advocate of teachers' noticing when students need them. Some Iyengar teachers say, 'Okay, everybody: four blankets.' But there are a number of people who don't need that. In the same way, the instruction that Shoulder Stand is not correct until you are completely vertical with your pelvis over your shoulders may not be correct for you. People can walk around with neck pain for long periods of time from doing the pose 'right.' I have noticed that people who need to do more of a Half Shoulder Stand, with their hips back a bit, can, if they stick with it over a number of months, get more vertical.

"In Plow or Half Shoulder Stand try lifting your chin, bringing your shoulders closer to your ears, and then releasing your chin again. Those two actions can help get the cervical spine off the floor. And as you gradually come more and more vertical in this position, notice how your neck feels, whether you are starting to strain it. Notice how it feels when you come down, and how it feels the next day. To push yourself into the 'right' version of the pose when your anatomy won't support it is not intelligent."

a friend turned her on to Paramahansa Yogananda's *Autobiography of a Yogi* and to *Yoga, Youth and Reincarnation,* one of the few books then in print that presented posture illustration alongside other aspects of yoga. For Patricia, it was like finding an instruction manual for equipment she was already using.

"I know this sounds weird, but by that time I had spontaneously begun doing poses," she says.

"In the mid-to-late sixties, there was just a lot of yoga floating around in the air. When I was coming down from acid or marijuana, my body would get very uncomfortable and I would automatically start stretching and then moving into postures like Full Lotus and Headstand." The practice became increasingly central in her life, even as she began studying to support herself as a dental hygienist. And in what Patricia now sees as a surprisingly

Practicing Plow/Shoulder Stand
Halasana/Salamba Sarvangasana

1. Bring your legs up and overhead into the Shoulder Stand preparation called Plow, as Patricia is demonstrating. In Plow, as in Shoulder Stand, you should feel the natural C curve in your cervical spine when you are in the pose. So if the back of your neck is jammed into the floor, work with a folded blanket or mat under your shoulders ❶. It is as important here as in Upward-Facing Bow preparation (p. 131) to roll the shoulders under the body. Use a strap if necessary to maintain external rotation and parallel alignment in your upper arms. If your feet do not reach the floor, press them into a block or rest your legs on a chair seat.

2. Once your Plow is well established, move into *Salamba Sarvangasana* ❷ by bending your elbows, placing your hands on your lower back, and lifting up one leg and then the other.

165

Plow/Shoulder Stand *(Halasana/Salamba Sarvangasana)*

significant way, her mother unwittingly encouraged the dicier of the two career options.

On a visit to Japan, where her father was next stationed, Patricia started showing her mother some yoga poses. "Where she got this idea I don't know—the wisdom of Mother, you know—but she said, 'I've heard you can hurt yourself with this stuff unless you have a teacher. Why don't you go find a teacher?' And she gave me $20, which bought a series of ten yoga classes in those days."

Back in Hawaii, Patricia started studying with a woman named Geri Aquino, who at that time taught what she recalls as the "devotional, gentle, sweet practices" of Swami Satchidananda's Integral Yoga. When Aquino relocated to northern California, Patricia continued to practice on her own, and began teaching what she knew to other students of yoga.

What she knew was altered radically by her first encounter with Iyengar, through the demonstration she watched in Tilden Park and through the two Bay-area classes he conducted afterward. "It scared me—but it also excited me and then made me want to look further," she says. At that point Patricia had moved to California and was apprenticing with her former teacher from Hawaii, who had became involved with the group that later came to found the San Francisco Iyengar Yoga Institute. As Patricia's own affiliation deepened, she took her first trip to India to study with

3. Using the wall is an excellent way to access the alignment principles that are key to this pose. Begin by lying on your back with your legs up the wall ③. End here if you are menstruating or if Shoulder Stand is contraindicated by a cervical spine injury or by overweight. In supporting your legs, which carry you around all day, this lovely semi-inversion relays the essence of peaceful surrender that is essential to yoga practice and especially critical for American practitioners to cultivate.

4. To move into Shoulder Stand, bend your knees just enough so that your feet come flat against the wall ④. Press into your feet to raise your hips until your knees are directly above your shoulders ⑤. (Again, use padding if your neck is grinding into the floor.) Roll your shoulders under one by one, then bend your elbows and place your palms on your lower back and extend one leg straight up to the ceiling ⑥. Keep your knees together and feel the vertical alignment here before you lift the other leg up to meet it ⑦.

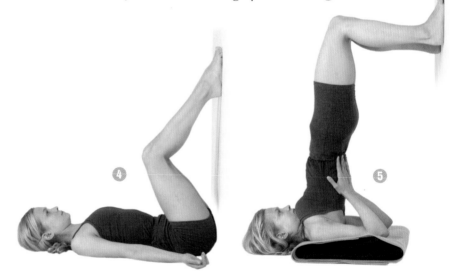

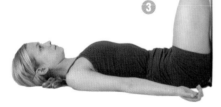

Iyengar in 1980. The experience was a "real eye-opener," she says.

"There was something more I wanted from yoga, which became apparent to me on that trip," she says. "You look around in India and you see there's a lot more to it: the devotional and meditative aspects I was not finding in the Iyengar training." Still, Patricia continued to study and teach the system as a faculty member at the San Francisco Iyengar Yoga Institute from 1987 through 1999.

The wisdom she acquired there still broadcasts in her teaching. "Such care and attention to detail tends to help people become more friendly with and at home in their body, and that understand-ing makes you more self-sufficient—which is extremely important," she says. "But the strong emphasis on the physical practice just didn't help me to open in places where I needed to open. It didn't help me to look deeper where I needed to look deeper. Yoga is when the mind ceases to identify itself with its vacillations, and theoretically you can arrive at it through asana practice alone. But there are eight limbs for a reason."

Students of B.K.S. Iyengar invariably recall that he brought up the eightfold path to yoga quickly and often. But for Patricia, his instruction in that regard "fell on deaf ears. There is something in my psychological makeup, I guess, that made it so all I could focus on was the sense of intimidation

5. Half Shoulder Stand 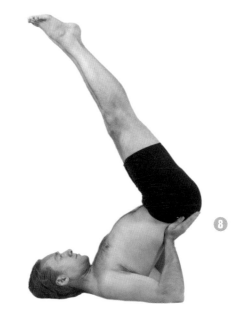, the standard version of the pose in the Viniyoga tradition, may be appropriate for you if you are stiff in the shoulders, neck, and upper back, or if your neck is uncomfortable in the more vertical alignment.

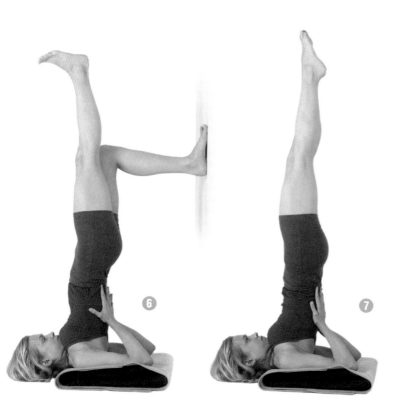

his presence brought to me," she says. "I kept trying to win his approval by doing the poses ever more to his satisfaction, which of course you could never do. What helped me to move away from that particular way of working was seeing myself in a photograph with Mr. Iyengar and seeing the pain in my face, the fear. And when I saw the picture I burst out into tears and I just thought, This is not the way for me."

In 1983, Patricia met Ed Brown, a devotee of Zen Buddhism, at a yoga class he regularly attended taught by Judith Lasater. "I would stay after the intermediate class to assist in her second class," Patricia says. "And in the fifteen minutes between classes, I would chat with Ed from time to time." Within a year the two had gotten together, and by 1988 they were teaching together.

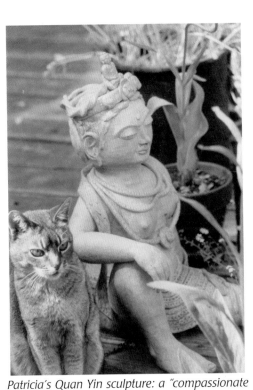

Patricia's Quan Yin sculpture: a "compassionate presence" that leads to her studio.

"At first it was, 'I'll do the yoga and you do the Zen, and never the twain shall meet,'" she says. "But over the years we discovered the commonality, amid all the differences, of the Hindu versus Buddhist teachings. Buddha was a yogi—that's pretty much acknowledged these days—and Buddhism and yoga come from the same root. The point is the same: to realize our true nature, through whatever practices appeal to you."

The mantra-style meditation Patricia had tried as a nineteen-year-old had not appealed to her as the postures did. And meditation as a practice was not encouraged in the Iyengar School. "Mr. Iyengar never had us sit down just to sit," she says. "He speaks very eloquently about how meditation can be experienced in any moment—in asana, in

breath work, in any other practice of the limbs. But if we were sitting, we were always working on our posture or on *pranayama.* It was never, 'Okay, now let the *pranayama* go.' So for me to go into the zendo, the Zen meditation hall, and just sit down and not be constantly having to correct myself, just to follow my breath as the path into concentration and deeper awareness was tremendously liberating."

That level of awareness continues to bring great texture to Patricia's yoga practice and to her teaching, which encompasses explorations like the one she taught to an assemblage of yoga teachers in August 2001. "If I ask you to take your attention to your hands," she posited, "notice that your attention goes more toward one than the other. Which one is it? Attend to the sensations in the one hand: the pulsation there, the quality of liquid always present within the body, whether it feels warm. Notice its size. If you're attending to a particular part of your body, you may find that its size in your awareness is different. Now see if you could draw your awareness to your other hand. Where the mind goes, so goes life force, or *prana.* So as you attend to getting your awareness and your life force in your non-dominant-side hand, you may find it increases in size—if not literally, in your sensorial experience. It starts to feel bigger, warmer, you may feel more pulsation sensations that maybe aren't there until you really attend to them. *Prana* and mind travel together, and the breath tags along. So that's why I just don't talk about anatomical correctness of the pose; I try to get people to experience that connection of life force and awareness and attention and how powerful that is."

Such cross-disciplinary influences are visible in Patricia's art, too. The representational and abstract sculptures of asana she used to craft are gradually being outnumbered by pieces on the order of the Quan Yin—the Chinese version of Buddhist Bodhisattva of compassion—that greets practitioners at the entrance to her studio. "The sculptures are either Hindu or Buddhist deities, but I don't follow all the iconography that the Buddhist and Hindu people do," Patricia says. "Anybody who has seen a Quan Yin recognizes it because of the position she is in. But it's like my personal version." Personal it may be, but Patricia's sculpture, like her teaching, tells the story of American yoga.

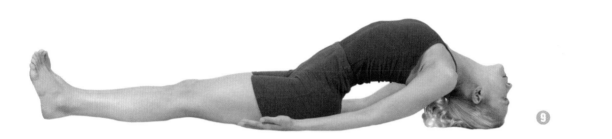

6. The classic counterpose to Shoulder Stand is Fish ⑨. But the Viniyoga tradition sees that as too jarring a transition for the cervical spine and recommends *Salabasana* instead ⑩.

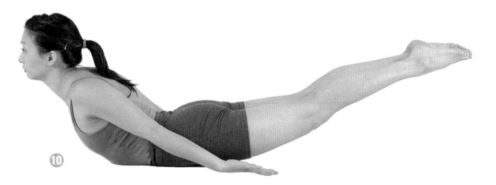

7. Advanced practitioners may choose to move from Shoulder Stand into a version of Fish that gives an intense stretch to the quadriceps and psoas muscles, not to mention the toes ⑪. From Shoulder Stand, move toward a reverse Plow by dropping your feet toward your buttocks and finally to the floor into Bridge pose, with the hands still supporting the lower back. From there, lift your heels, tiptoe your feet together and back until they rest under your buttocks, and take hold of your ankles. Reach your arms overhead in a prayer and breathe as fully and calmly as you do in Fish.

David Life
Fish
(Matsyasana)

For David Life the route to yoga began with asana. Postures take him there still, on a daily basis, and he's adamant about why that is. "Asana is not just a preparation for what you're going to do, which is physical," he says. "It's what techniques do you use in asana to lessen the attachment to the physical body and to increase the attachment to the subtle or spiritual body."

At Jivamukti Yoga Center in New York, the school David has run since 1989 along with his partner, Sharon Gannon, the tenet of asana as a spiritual practice is palpable. The very walls throb with it, as students lift and press through the school's vigorous brand of Vinyasa Yoga, or what in the case of Jivamukti is better described as *vinyasa svadhyaya*, or progressive Self-study. "Asana practice works in conjunction with meditation and breath awareness to purify your mind so you can have this transcendental experience," David says. "And when done in synchrony with the other techniques, it can bring you to enlightenment."

He didn't always feel that way. On the heels of his thirtieth birthday David went to a yoga class—largely because he wanted to spend more time with Sharon, whom he had met when her musical group performed at his East Village café. As an enthusiastic new

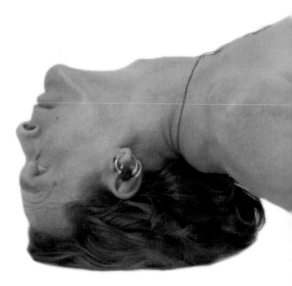

THE YOGA OF THE POSE: "In *Matsyasana,* the heart is higher than any other part of the body. It's the only posture that puts the heart above everything else. And that's a metaphor for what we're trying to do in the practice, which is to balance the intuitive and rational aspects of being. Since the heart is so underplayed, to let it break out to the top level of the body and be the most important, prominent thing is symbolically potent. Some people go too much that way. They become anti-intellectual—everything is about feeling— and that's taking it too far in the other direction. As a yogi, you want balance. But our heart is kind of stifled, so sometimes you have to emphasize the feeling aspect more so you are not afraid to express it.

"On a physical level, of course, it's used as a counterpose for Shoulder Stand and Plow, because it opens the base of the throat and the heart center to a flow of energy that was closed off by the chin lock. And it's an easy, safe beginning backbend in that it tones the back of the body and creates openness of the front of the body."

HOW STUDENTS COMMONLY MISS IT: "By shrugging their shoulders, allowing the upper chest to be caved in a bit as they do it. By not activating the back of the body enough to pull the spine in toward the center of the body. And if the front of the body is locked and won't open up because you are stubbornly holding onto fear, anxiety, or anger, you can miss it."

HOW TO MAKE SURE YOU CONNECT: "I think that's all about intention and visualization. If your intention is clearly to dedicate your efforts to the well-being of others, there's nothing you can do that would selfishly inhibit that movement. I like to visualize fish when I'm doing it. My favorite visualization is a porpoise leaping out of the water, a vision of leaping in pure joy. I let that inspire me to do my little fish thing there, which hardly compares, but I use that vision for inspiration.

"Once a student told me that when she comes out of Fish, she gets spasms in her lower back. So I suggested that when she gets into it, she lift her seat and move her tailbone toward the seat to lengthen the lower back, and then reemphasize the opening of the chest and upper back. She said that helped. You don't think of Fish as a lower-back impacting backbend, but if you're doing it unconsciously, it could be.

"People who tighten against the pose should lie on something—a bolster, a pillow— and do passive opening. Support the head so the neck isn't in an extreme position and use a block or bolster to let the chest expand. Then just lie on that for some duration so that the fear ebbs away."

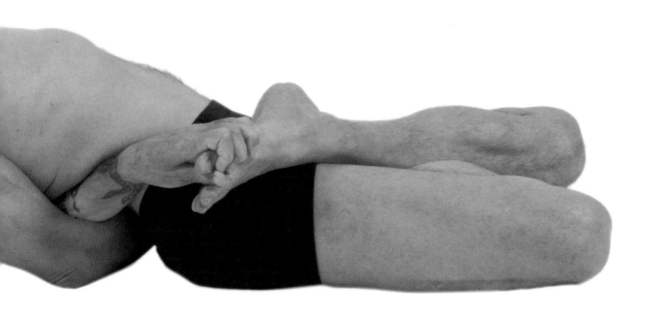

Fish *(Matsyasana)*

practitioner, Sharon was attending class frequently, but David's first experience left him "a bit overwhelmed. I could barely wait to get back outside and smoke a cigarette," he recalls. Subsequent classes moved him to tears, however—and not because of nicotine withdrawal. "It was upsetting my whole world. I'm sure everybody goes through that to some degree when they begin to see that this is not a workout, but a workshop where your whole psychology is laid out on the table. At first that's scary, to see all of your shadows. But then you start to learn that you can rearrange them—throw a couple out, make a couple bigger, and then get past them to move toward a deeper awareness."

The premise wasn't entirely new to David. As a child of the '60s, he'd become familiar with higher states of consciousness but had found no sustainable way to achieve them. A painter before he came to yoga, he leaned toward visionary and mystical subjects. His taste in literature ran to Yeats, Allen Ginsberg, and Gary Snyder. "I didn't want to just scratch the surface in this lifetime. When I began practicing yoga, I saw that it all pulled together, that these were techniques for reaching the ecstatic states the great artists and philosophers talked about."

He and Sharon began doing intense *sadhana,*

Practicing Fish
(Matsyasana)

1. Lie down on your back and prop yourself up on your elbows ❶. On an inhale, arch your entire spine and let your head fall back. As you exhale, walk your hands toward your heels until the crown of your head rests on the floor ❷. If you are comfortable here, you can work on building strength in this pose by lifting your legs 45 degrees off the floor and extending the arms, palms together, fingers pointing toward the toes ❸.

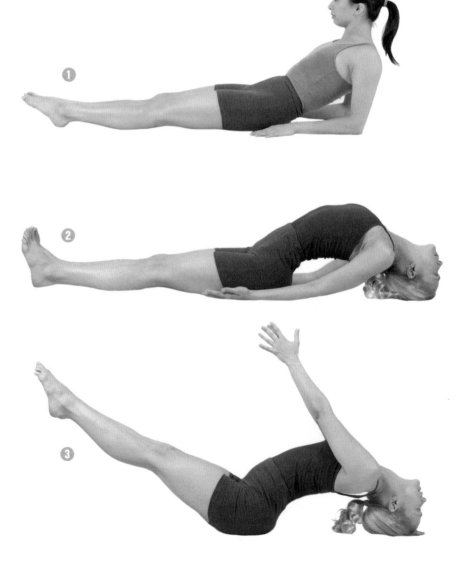

2. For the Sivananda-style Fish ④, wriggle your elbows and forearms beneath you, slide the palms facedown under your seat, and arch into the pose from there. Take care, however, that this approach doesn't cause you to hunch your shoulders toward your ears and crimp your neck—one reason some teachers eschew the variation.

3. If Fish is difficult for you, try lying on a block or a bolster to allow expansion across the chest ⑤. Turn the block up a notch to deepen into the backbend ⑥, or prop your head up on a towel or blanket if it is too intense.

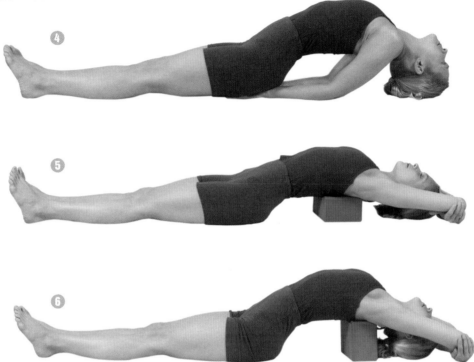

or practice, in New York City. They regularly bicycled up to the Sivananda center in the morning, over to Dharma Mittra or Swami Bua's studio a little later in the day, and back downtown for class with their original hatha yoga teacher at night. David's increasingly single-minded pursuit led him eventually to India. He initially took teacher training at the Sivananda ashram in Kerala, then went repeatedly for study with the Astanga Yoga master K. Pattabhi Jois, as well as with the reclusive Swami Nirmalananda.

Nirmalananda, known as the Anarchist Swami, had in earlier years traveled the world and met with foreign dignitaries to promote world peace. After four years of his tutelage, David asked his guru for a mantra initiation, but Nirmalananda decided to initiate him as a monk in the Order of Sannyasa. "At first I thought, 'Are you crazy?' but

he was my guru and I recognized that I was being given a gift."

Once back in New York, David found certain of the vows more difficult to maintain than in India. Swamis are meant to live on what grace provides, "but being homeless in New York makes it hard to teach yoga," he notes. Nirmalananda agreed that he could have a modest apartment and keep a small bank account. On his initiation, David had been given two sets of the traditional unsewn, hand-dyed clothes, with ocher stones. "You have to rinse the clothes in cold water and hang dry them every other day so that the ocher stone stays," David says. "I wrote to say, 'You know, Swami, this ocher thing just isn't working out.'" His guru gave him permission to wear sewn, dyed clothes. "The Gap was running a sale on orange clothes and I got everything orange. The

Fish (Matsyasana)

neighbors called me Orange Man."

Over the next two and a half years, David found that being a swami was making it increasingly difficult to live simply as a yogi. He was attracting a more troublesome sort of attention among his students, the very sort that monkhood is meant to deflect. He decided to renounce his vows. "Nirmalananda was disappointed but gracious. He told me, 'Sannyasa is not in your clothes or your bank account; it's inside. As far as I'm concerned, you'll always be Sannyasa.'"

Berobed or not, David began using all the hues from his broadening palette of influences to convey the essence of his teachings. Standing on your head during one of his classes, you're as like-

ly to hear a recorded lecture by Ram Dass or Alan Watts as you are to receive detailed posture instruction. And if you are taken aback by a hip-hop track during Sun Salutations, there's no sense getting in a funk over it, since Mozart could well be waiting in the wings. David bookends his classes with readings from or references to the sutras or the Upanishads or whatever has been on his mind. And it's all interesting and intelligent because he is interesting and intelligent.

"I think the key for the development of yoga in the West is the proper integration of the ancient with a modern translation," David says. "And that's happening—whether we want it to or not. It's a testimonial to the universality and timelessness of

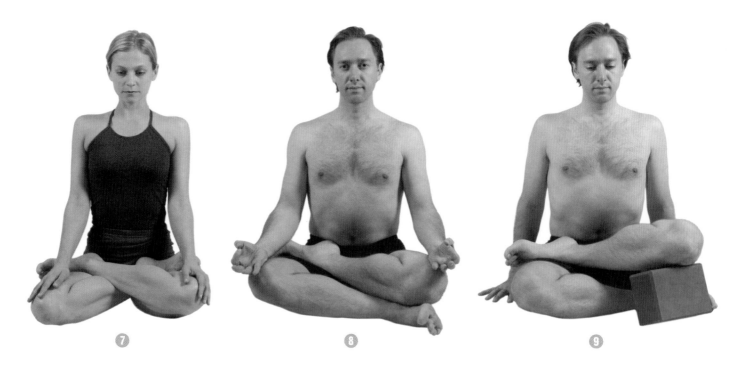

4. The advanced *Matsyasana* variation David Life is demonstrating includes Bound Lotus Pose, or *Baddha Padmasana*. If you are like the majority of Americans, arriving at Lotus ❼ or even Half-Lotus ❽ takes progressive effort. But the inquiry is one worth making, David says. "A yogi can't settle for, 'Oh, my muscles are tight,' and not deal with the underlying cause. So work with padding ❾, but also feel more and think less. Stop analyzing. See how long you can just count the

breaths and not label your experience as good or bad or difficult or easy, but just remain neutral in the midst of it. Slowly and carefully begin to know the difference between an intense feeling and a bad feeling. To transcend an intense feeling doesn't mean pushing past it in a physical sense. Just let it be intense and change your mind about how it affects you. You can witness it just like you witness the thinking process until you don't get so tangled up in it."

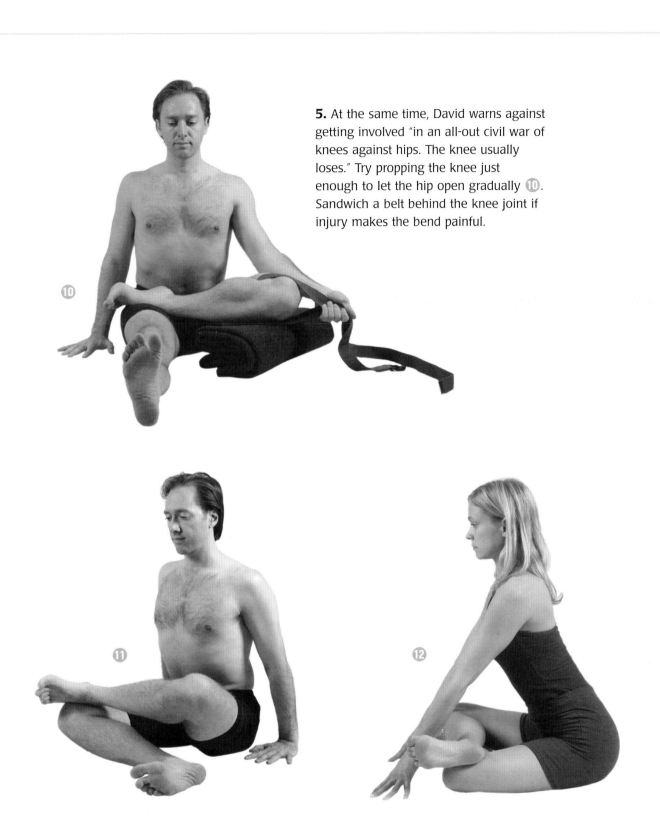

5. At the same time, David warns against getting involved "in an all-out civil war of knees against hips. The knee usually loses." Try propping the knee just enough to let the hip open gradually ⑩. Sandwich a belt behind the knee joint if injury makes the bend painful.

6. As an approach to *Padmasana*, Rodney Yee swears by the efficacy of Ankle-to-Knee pose ⑪. Stack your ankles and knees directly atop each other, making a box with your legs. Place your palms on the floor alongside your hips, sit tall, close your eyes, and send deep, calm breaths into areas of retention. Inhale and accept them for what they are; exhale and let them change. If you are reasonably comfortable here, place your fingertips in front of your shins ⑫ and walk yourself into a forward bend.

yoga. If you keep the essential aspects intact and let them shape themselves into the present moment the way they should, then it works. We don't want to lose the validity of the teachings when we present our Western take on them, which we have to. We aren't living in the India of two centuries ago."

It was right in their own backyard, or a few miles north of it, that David and Sharon came upon another of their gurus: Sri Brahmananda Sarasvati, who founded the Yoga Society of New York in 1964. Back then virtually every major yogi passing through the East Coast stopped at his Ananda Ashram in Monroe, New York. To this day it remains a serene outpost of spiritual practice, led by the remnants of the community that sprang

WE ARE WHAT WE EAT

Most Americans consider vegetarianism, which is part and parcel of the yogic precept of *ahimsa* (nonviolence), an alternative lifestyle choice. But in a culture known for conspicuous consumption, the practice of conscious eating is fast becoming a biological imperative. Studies now confirm what fishermen everywhere already know: The oceans' fish are disappearing. Mass production of the inexpensive meat Westerners consider their due has begun to sicken us, as it does the animals we consume. And so-called factory farming is devastating to the environment. One of the people campaigning most actively to redress these unsustainable trends is a man who stood to gain from them.

In the late 1960s John Robbins turned his back on the Baskin-Robbins ice-cream fortune created by his father, whose "31 Flavors" and successful franchising turned the little stores into big business. "In a world where a child dies of hunger every two seconds while elsewhere abundant resources are going to waste, adding a thirty-second flavor just didn't seem like an adequate response," John says. The agribusiness techniques he witnessed then seem relatively benign compared to today's. "You don't have to be a yogi, a vegetarian, or an animal rights activist"—John is all three—"to be appalled by the level of cruelty that is standard operating procedure in commercial dairies and feedlots."

No matter how you slice it, the foods produced through these methods are of dubious benefit. The FDA says the use of bovine growth hormone to increase milk production has no ill

effects on humans. But E. coli in undercooked beef is not acceptable in anyone's book. "Cows are herbivores, and E. coli hardly exists in grass-fed cows," John says. "But when you feed them grain, which is cheaper for the industry, it wreaks havoc on their digestive systems and creates breeding grounds for the bacteria," John says. "Since the animals are crammed together and standing in their feces, the bacteria spread quickly." Farm-raised fish like salmon are developing new diseases, for which they, like livestock, are treated with antibiotics. And the caged fish no longer contain highly nutritional omega-3 fatty acids, since they do not eat the algae that produce it.

As John states in his books and in addresses to organizations from the United Nations to Oxfam, a ten percent reduction in America's beef consumption would save twelve million tons of grain annually—enough to alleviate hunger or hunger-caused disease worldwide. That grain might not reach the world's hungry, he allows, "but there's one guarantee: It will not reach them if we eat it ourselves by cycling it through the animals we consume.

"I'm not trying to say what is right or wrong for all people in all situations. But developing yogic consciousness helps us realize that what we do to the planet, to other animals, and to people who are less fortunate than ourselves we do to ourselves. We must begin to make choices toward a sustainable, humane approach to existence. And moving away from eating factory farm animal products is a big piece of that."

up around the Indian yogi. Although Saraswati died in 1993, shortly after Sharon and David met him, his teachings continue to have a major influence on them and their work, including their emphasis on the recitation of Sanskrit.

David often begins his classes with what in the Sivananda tradition is called the Guru Brahma chant: *guru brahma, guru vishnu, guru devo maheshwara, guru sakshat, param brahma, tasmai sri gurave namaha.* He explains that chanting it with sincere understanding makes us cognizant of the myriad teachers in one's life and of the teacher that life is—that it is all fodder for Self-realization. And although external teachers are paramount, "the obligation of a yoga teacher is to be a guru. If they are not being gurus, they should call themselves physical education instructors." David reminds students again and again that the inner teacher is where it's at.

"People ask me if I was confused having three gurus, and I always say no, because I was only perceiving one guru. It appears in many bodies over time in many eras, but there's only one guru. Anyone who thinks they are seeing many gurus needs to practice *pratyahara,* which is the practice of seeing the one in the many. When they have that perfected, they will no longer be confused.

"The guru is your Self," he says. "You should not be dependent on anyone outside of you to 'do it' to you, even as you come to rely on teachers of great knowledge and insight. Yoga practice can't just be a hedonistic, self-centered activity. The Self exists wherever you look, so if you are not seeing it wherever you're looking, you need to heighten your perception."

In encouraging people to do just that, David takes his position as an increasingly public figure extremely seriously. He and Sharon have always used their teaching as a platform for political activism, addressing issues they consider critical

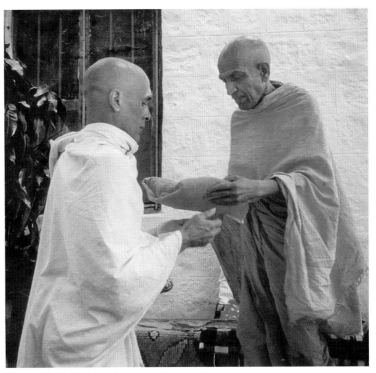
David being initiated into the Order of Sannyasa by Swami Nirmalananda in 1989.

to the pursuit of liberation for all beings. High on the list is vegetarianism, which he teaches like an asana. "For me the yoga techniques are a kind of empty slate you can fill with whatever you want," he says. "You can fill it with just breath consciousness; you can fill it with self-centeredness; you can fill it with compassion and awareness and supreme consciousness. One of a yoga teacher's chief jobs is to enable people to fill that space with consciousness.

"The things I talk about are ways to address commonly held ideas in our culture about how we live and why we're here—and to question them. In yoga asana practice your consciousness and brain chemistry are altered. So when you hear these ideas and music and words in that state of heightened awareness, your energetic body is affected. Over time it becomes an energetic body that's in harmony with these great ideas of nonharming, selflessness, consciousness-raising. That's why I introduce catalysts for change into my yoga classes—because I have to."

Nischala Joy Devi
Corpse Pose
(Savasana)

After thirty years of teaching yoga in America, Nischala Joy Devi has arrived at a subtle redefinition of asana. The usual translation of the directive *sthira-sukham-asanam*, as posited in Patanjali's *Yoga Sutras* two millennia ago, is that posture should be steady and comfortable. NischalaDevi's gentle twist on the sutra—"Asana is steadiness of the body that expresses the natural comfort and happiness of our being"—epitomizes her teachings. So does the way she has softened into her role as a powerful healer.

In her early twenties NischalaDevi became dissatisfied with the contribution she was making as a physician's assistant in her hometown of Philadelphia. "As I watched bodies die, I began to realize that we are much more than the body," she says. She left medicine to find out what that "much more" might be.

It was the late 1960s, a time when a whole generation of young Americans were to varying degrees joined in that self-same pursuit. Backpacking her way across country and living "close to nature," NischalaDevi wound up taking a yoga class in Denver with a teacher who "showed me the scope of yoga, how deep you can get," she recalls. "It took me back to a place I knew as a child, when I would meditate without knowing what meditation was." Then, at the Integral Yoga Institute in San Francisco in 1973, NischalaDevi saw a photograph of Swami Satchidananda and was instantly drawn to him. "I knew he

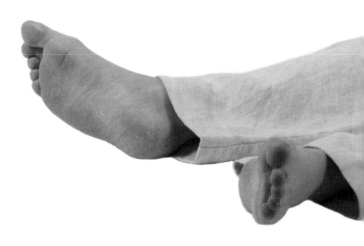

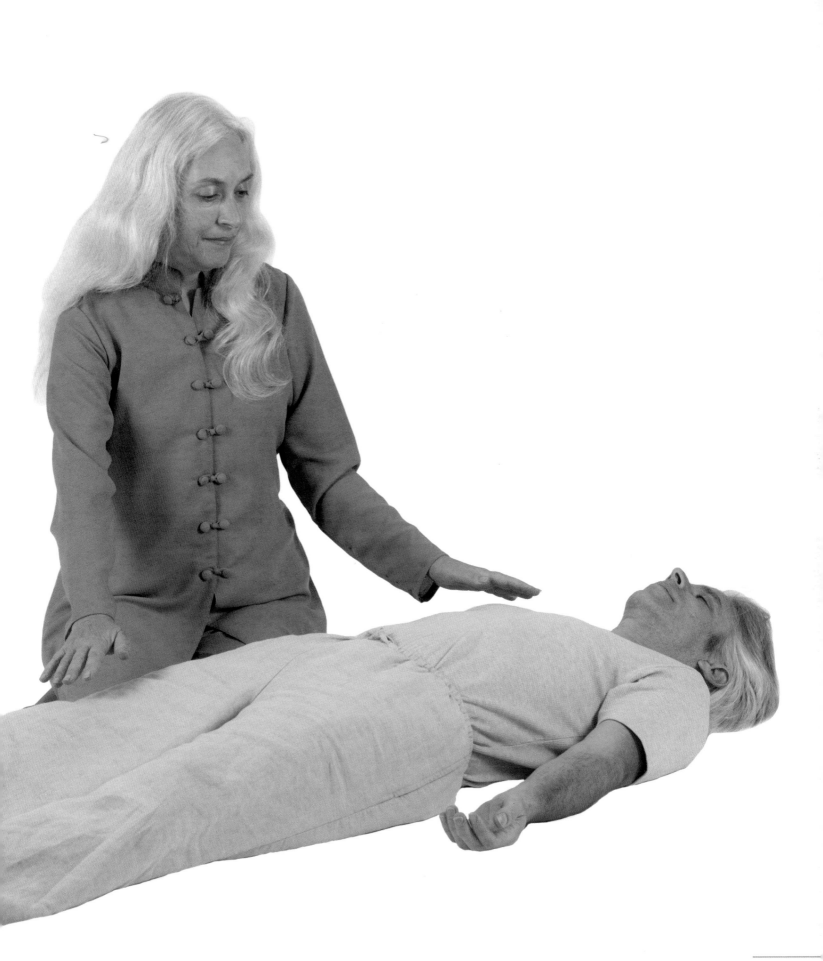

Corpse Pose *(Savasana)*

THE YOGA OF THE POSE: *"Savasana* is the physical asana, but what you do with your mind changes it to deep relaxation, which guides you to deeper levels of consciousness. Most people who do asana cannot abandon their body; they are totally with it, in pleasant or unpleasant situations. One of the first steps to deep relaxation, which can take people months to learn how to do, is to let go of the body and then to let go of the mind. Then when you go back to do asana again, you know what if feels like to really let go."

HOW STUDENTS COMMONLY MISS IT: "People don't take the time to do it. They think nothing is happening when they're lying there. So they cut that part short, without realizing that more happens in stillness than at any other time. And people who say, 'I don't want to just lie there for fifteen, twenty minutes. I have things to do!'—they're the ones who need it most."

HOW TO MAKE SURE YOU CONNECT: "Do it first and do it afterward, and cut back on the asana if you have to. I even suggest people do it as a separate practice—when you come home, in the middle of the day, in your office—because it's such an important practice, and it becomes more and more important as life becomes more and more stressful. Systematic relaxation calms the mind. This is a *pratyahara* (p. 56); it becomes the step before *dharana* and before meditation."

NischalaDevi's method for deepest relaxation moves systematically through the *maya koshas*, the energetic layers that ensheathe our essence. "For people whose minds are racing, this is perfect because it starts with the body and then goes to the vital energy, the *prana*, and then finally it gets to the mind and emotions," she says. "And by that time the mind is calmed, and you move deeper and deeper into your true nature."

could help me find the joy I wanted to experience," she says. Hunch became fact when she took a class with the man she came to call her guru.

"He had a great sense of humor and depth to his teaching," NischalaDevi says. "And he understood the completeness of yoga. He called his organization Integral Yoga because it integrated all the aspects: the devotional, the psychological, the intellectual path, the service. And it meant integration not only within the yoga but within the world, which was very important to me."

After four years of studying with Swami Satchidananda, she took her monastic vows and became a *sannyasin,* or swami. Half of the swamis in the Integral Yoga organization were female. In this as in most things—including the directive to take yoga to the West—Swami Satchidananda took his cue from his guru, Swami Sivananda, who

had initiated women into the monastic order in India at a time when their inclusion was virtually unheard of.

Over the next sixteen years NischalaDevi lived and taught at Integral Yoga Institutes around the country, serving as director in Los Angeles and in Denver. As the director of teacher training for the entire organization, she helped develop its basic and advanced teacher training programs.

"For us asana is a more gentle form. Its purpose is to strengthen the body for meditation—not as a practice unto itself—so that when the energies of higher consciousness start to move through, the body is strong enough to hold them. Class started with meditation and chanting, then asana, then deep relaxation for fifteen minutes or more, then *pranayama* and meditation and peace chants at the end for closing. In an hour-and-fifteen-minute class there was only half an hour of

Practicing Corpse Pose *(Savasana)*

At the close of asana practice lie on your back and take a moment to make yourself comfortable. If you have lower back pain, you might find it helpful to place a rolled blanket or mat under your knees. If you have an exaggerated C curve at the back of the neck and your chin tips up to the ceiling, rest your head on a folded towel or blanket. An eye pillow can deepen relaxation by blocking light and involuntary eye movements. At the very least, be certain that you are warm.

Make whatever final motions you need to make, then stop moving. Arrange your legs mat-width or so apart and lay your arms a few inches from your body. Turn your palms faceup in a gesture of receptivity and surrender. Soften your brow. Let your face be the face you had before you were born.

Great teachers take you through *Savasana* in different ways. Sivananda instructors employ a lullingly methodical script of autosuggestion that you are encouraged to repeat mentally: *I relax my ankles and feet, I relax my ankles and feet, my ankles and feet are relaxed. I relax my calves, knees, and thighs. . . .* Some teachers play music or chant for their students. Others say nothing at all. Regardless of their approach, "get really good at this one," Erich Schiffmann advises. Afford yourself the profundity of this posture, in which the yogi comes to know death in order to understand life.

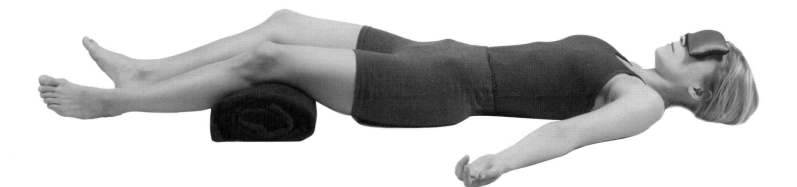

asana." The format, like the training, is essentially the same today.

NischalaDevi renounced her formal vows in 1991—"I went into the ashram to be free, and I left the ashram to be free," she notes—but she has never relinquished what she calls her eternal commitment. That pledge deepened through her marriage four years later to Bhaskar Deva, another longtime monk in the Satchidananda organization. "We feel that we are still living those vows of selfless service," she says. "To be able to give to another person and to humanity at the same time—that to me is real spirituality. If I put the ocher robes back on, it doesn't mean I would change who I am; I didn't change when I took them off. *Sannyasin* is about bringing yourself to a higher level of consciousness as a means to serve humanity."

NischalaDevi had begun doing that quite concretely in 1982. In that year two long-time Integral students, Dean Ornish, M.D., then a young Harvard medical resident, and Michael Lerner, Ph.D., each wanted to bring yoga's benefits to bear on heart disease and cancer, their respective fields of specialization. They turned to NischalaDevi to help them do it. The results proved nothing short of revolutionary, both in the Commonweal Cancer Help Program and in the medical study that produced Dr. Ornish's Program for Reversing Heart Disease.

When medical studies corroborated Dr. Ornish's claim that coronary heart disease can be reversed through a low-fat vegetarian diet combined with yoga and meditation, ten hospitals nationwide opted to adopt his program. Dr. Ornish

---

PERMEATING EASE: THE MAYA KOSHAS

STAGE 1 (*anna maya kosha:* the food or physical body): Begin by relaxing the body with the body. After arranging yourself comfortably on your back, systematically tighten then release each foot and leg, your buttocks, your abdomen, each arm and hand, your shoulders, your neck, head, and face. Move consciously and slowly, pausing after each part to notice how you feel.

STAGE 2 (*prana maya kosha:* the breath or vital body): In the same deliberate, systematic way begin relaxing the body with the breath. Inhale deeply, and as you exhale, send the breath to your legs and feet. Allow them to relax. As you move through the entire body in this way, get specific: Inhale deeply and exhale into each toe, your ankles, your calves, your knees and thighs, the backs of your eyes, your heart—everywhere the breath can reach.

STAGE 3 (*mano maya kosha:* the mind and senses): Now use the mind and the senses to relax the body. Notice how still the breath has become. Then brush every inch of your body with this gentle breath "to remove any subtle tension, thoughts, feelings, or memories," Nischala Joy Devi recommends. Guide the breath from your feet to your jaw to the hairs on your head.

STAGE 4 (*vijnana maya kosha:* the intuition or seat of higher wisdom): Allow your higher wisdom to move to the fore by bringing awareness to the entrance and exit of the gentle breath. Invite healing energy on each inhale and, as if from a distance, feel yourself let go of thoughts, feelings, and tension as you exhale.

STAGE 5 (*ananda maya kosha:* the bliss body): Here we meld with the wisdom we have relaxed into by letting ourselves know what we have always known: This is who we are.

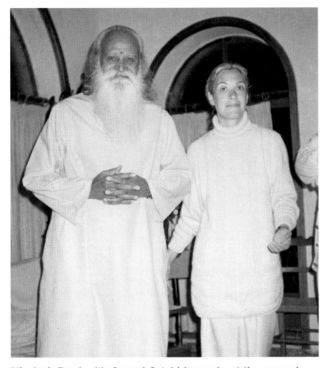

NischalaDevi *with Swami Satchidananda at the annual European Union Federation of Yoga Teachers meeting in Zinal, Switzerland, in 1988.*

once again hired NischalaDevi to aid in its implementation. She selected and trained teachers to administer the program, which came to accommodate deeper and deeper states of relaxation.

"It is very hard for most people to meditate, but with good relaxation first they can," NischalaDevi says. "And there is documented evidence that when patients do more of the yoga and meditation portion, they get better faster." The study is currently being replicated at the Walter Reed Army Medical Center, with similar results.

The application of yoga's benefits continues to drive NischalaDevi's work. "People with life-threatening diseases generally come to me not with the thought of realizing their true self through yoga, but because they're facing death or surgery," she says. "Unlike healthy people who can use their bodies to deepen their awareness, these people can't. So we take them past the body and move them right into the subtle aspects that allow them to heal." Her primary service now is training yoga teachers and healthcare professionals to share these practices with people who are ill. She calls it Yoga of the Heart.

"One of the things I teach is not just how to help people but how to have compassion. When people are ill, they are vulnerable, but they are also very open to knowing who they are. Healthcare professionals and yoga teachers can work to help people use illness as a tool for transformation, for leaping into a higher level of consciousness."

A Yoga of the Heart session is at its core what NischalaDevi has been practicing and teaching all her life. "Instead of chanting and meditation, I do a relaxation to begin with, about seven minutes with students on their backs. Next I take them through modified asana, and they do a very long, deep relaxation, fifteen to twenty minutes, moving through the *koshas*. Then they sit up and do *pranayama*, a little bit of guided imagery, and meditation to close."

For NischalaDevi Self-knowledge begins and ends with compassion. "Does disease come when the heart stops loving? Is it that simple? I think it's that simple," she says. "Through stress, people come to know that they're working too hard, that they're not eating right, that they're pushing themselves beyond. This allows us to be open for disease, because we're not taking care of who we are." Her antidote to this modern American pandemic is the peaceful pursuit of deep relaxation, afforded by well-practiced *Savasana,* or Corpse pose. "This is the pose that changes you," NischalaDevi reminds us sweetly. "And changing you changes the world."

Swami Srinivasananda
Shining Skull Breath Expansion
(Kapalabhati Pranayama)

In 1977 Swami Srinivasananda—or Mark Ashley, as he was then called—went searching for his teacher. Srinivasananda's quest toward peace had formally begun eight years earlier, when he approached draft age and the United States was at the height of the Vietnam War. The conscientious objector status he applied for required an exceptionally well-reasoned defense, and writing it served as his unofficial indoctrination into yoga philosophy. "It took me into deep questioning about who am I, what I am doing here, what is the purpose of life: questions yoga really deals with," Srinivasananda says.

At the University of California at Berkeley, Srinivasananda majored in rhetoric, which allowed him to study everything from poetry to politics. He also immersed himself in *Richard Hittleman's Yoga: 28 Day Exercise Plan* to continue the investigation of asanas he had begun in high school to correct his adolescent slouch. While his college studies helped him develop good critical writing skills and an understanding of constitutional law, Srinivasananda felt no strong pull toward a career in either field. "Critical writing had become difficult because I had reached a point where if I couldn't say anything positive, it wasn't worth saying," he recalls. "My idealism was challenged even at the legal aid center where I was working when the person in charge ran off with all the money."

After Berkeley, Srinivasananda took music and carpentry courses at a junior college, then gave everything up for a sojourn in the mountains, where he backpacked and meditated alone. It struck him that he needed a teacher, and he made a highly specific list of what he was looking for. The search would be fraught with temptations and pitfalls.

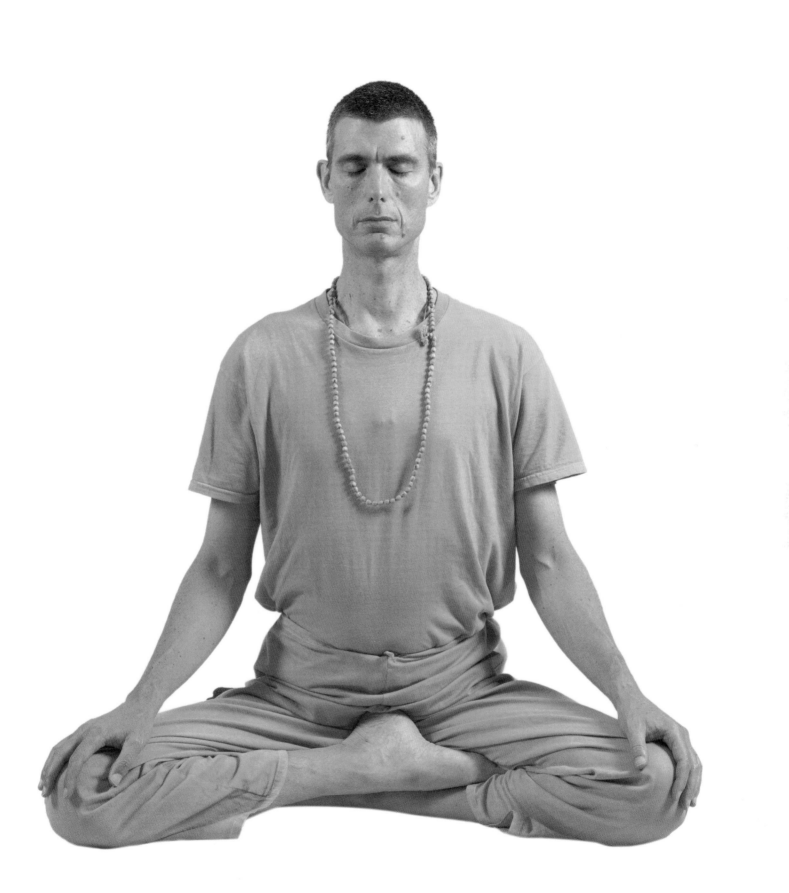

Shining Skull Breath Expansion *(Kapalabhati Pranayama)*

THE YOGA OF THE PRACTICE:
"I don't think there is a more direct way to expand life-force energy or *prana*—which is one definition of *pranayama*—than to work with *Kapalabhati*. It compels you to breathe diaphragmatically, which frees up tension held in the abdomen. If someone starts to get emotional, you tell them to breathe—but what you're telling them is to breathe diaphragmatically. A lot of emotional stress is created when the movement of the diaphragm is constricted. You cannot concentrate unless you have enough oxygen and enough breath.

"On a sheer physical level the purpose of breathing is to get more oxygen into your blood and brain, and to expel the unwanted gases. And *Kapalabhati* does that in a very focused and relaxed way, unlike jogging or intensive physical exercise, which generate more physical and mental stress.

"One of the beauties of *Kapalabhati* is that it teaches you to concentrate and to relax, which allows you to refine your awareness of *prana.* Then you become able to discern where you are holding tension and direct the *prana* there in a very conscious way during *kumbhaka*, or breath retention. So *Kapalabhati* serves as a foundation for more advanced *pranayama.*"

HOW STUDENTS COMMONLY MISS IT: "The biggest obstacle is when people engage in backward-breathing instead of breathing diaphragmatically. If the diaphragm moves in the wrong direction as you breathe—if you contract your abdomen while you inhale and release it while you exhale—this results in the negative physical and psychological effects of hyperventilation.

"Students are sometimes too forceful with *Kapalabhati,* which is not good for relaxation or for concentration. Another common mistake is incorrect posture. If you collapse as you sit, then you cannot breathe with the abdomen."

HOW TO MAKE SURE YOU CONNECT: "To learn *pranayama,* you must first learn to breathe correctly. Place your hand on your abdomen and feel it go out as you inhale and in as you exhale. If you have difficulty creating or sensing this movement, do the exercise lying down on your back. Become aware of any tension you are holding in your solar plexus, your chest, neck, and shoulders, and your heart. Releasing this type of rigidity can move you away from fear—especially irrational fear.

"Elevate your seat on a pillow or blanket if needed to make sure you are on your sitting bones as opposed to collapsing into your lower back. Draw your shoulders back and down and your spine straight up. If your head is jutting forward, bring it back and up. Let go of tension in your neck and face. It's not easy to relax your face when you first do *Kapalabhati,* but learning to do it really can change the way you hold your face in general. And it relaxes your mind.

"Relaxation and concentration are the key to all asana and *pranayama* practice. So during retention, you should hold the breath only as long as it is comfortable, just as you should go only as deep into an asana as you comfortably can. When people try to hold their breath too long, you can see the strain in their face, and the diaphragm will start to go up and down as they try not to swallow—which creates unwanted tension. The idea is to experience *prana,* and to experience *prana* is to experience grace—if the focus, the intention, and the devotion are there."

Srinivasananda decided to head north. His girlfriend at the time agreed to accompany him on his quest, and they crossed the border into Ontario in his VW bus. Thanks to their hippie attire and the erratic behavior of a hitchhiker they picked up along the way, Srinivasananda wound up in jail for a night on a marijuana possession charge. "It was a sobering experience, and I made a vow never to touch drugs again."

The police released Srinivasananda on condition that he leave the country within twenty-four hours. He dropped his now skittish girlfriend in Michigan and then turned around and drove right back across the border. "I felt like I was being led," he says. And so he was—in part by a mysterious traveler who directed him exactly where he wanted to go.

Srinivasananda met the traveler just as he arrived at a small Canadian version of the yearly hippie gathering called the Rainbow Festival. "I looked around at these old hippies who had been wandering for years, and all they could talk about were memories of times gone by," he says. "They were lost spirits, like an image out of *A Christmas Carol.* It struck me that if I continued in my wandering, this was where I would end up."

Srinivasananda says that it was a real blessing that he had such a clear idea of what he was looking for: "a place where I could study with a yoga master—someone who was not just hiding away, but who was politically aware and doing work in the world. I said I wanted to do asanas, speak French, engage in music, writing, and the practice of rituals, to work hard and not have to work for money, and to experience a real Canadian winter." The traveler said he knew a place just like that and gave Srinivasananda the address of the Sivananda ashram in Val Morin, Quebec.

Escaping the morose gathering of "lost spirits," Srinivasananda drove directly to Val Morin, where the engine of his VW bus petered out as soon as he passed through the ashram gate. "The director came out, and I told her I wanted to practice yoga, work, do chanting and maybe some writing. She told me they'd try me out for a month." In essence, he never left.

"I discovered that leading a disciplined life actually led to the freedom I had been searching for in my travels," he says. "The asanas and the rituals became part of an inner transformation, as did the practice of *brahmacharya,* or celibacy. Life in California was very loose in the '70s, and to be able to relate to women without having that sexual vibration was a wonderful liberation. Then I saw a picture of Swami Sivananda that matched the vision of the Swami who I had felt guiding me on this journey. It struck me that although he was no longer in a physical form, Swami Sivananda had led me to Swami Vishnu-devananda."

In addition to setting up twenty-five centers worldwide and establishing the first yoga teacher training course in America, Vishnu-devananda was a warrior for peace. From the time his guru, Swami Sivananda, had sent him to the West in 1957,

> "Wearing the ocher-colored cloth is necessary for one who has a changed mind. Due to the force of habit, when the senses move among the sense-objects, the moment you look at the colored cloth you wear it will remind you that you are a Sannyasin. It will give you a kick and save you from vicious actions. It has got its own glory and advantages. Only a real Sannyasin can cut off all connections and ties and completely get rid of attachment. The robe is of great service when one appears on the platform for preaching. Common people will easily receive ideas from a Sannyasin. Some hypocrites say: 'We have given coloring to our minds. We need not change the clothes.' I do not believe these men. Only those who have cravings, passions, and attachments, and who are timid, dread to change the cloth, and thus bring forth false, ingenious, unsound arguments." —Swami Sivananda

Shining Skull Breath Expansion *(Kapalabhati Pranayama)*

Vishnu-devananda actively embodied the ideal of *ahimsa,* or nonviolence. In 1969 he took off in a Piper Apache twin-engine plane painted by the pop artist Peter Max and flew himself around the world, disseminating his message of peace. In England he was joined by the actor Peter Sellers, with whom he flew to Belfast to distribute peace pamphlets and flowers to the British troops and the Irish Republican Army. When Swami Vishnu flew over the Suez Canal and Israeli fighter jets radioed orders to turn back, he replied that he had orders from higher up. (Imprisoned in Egypt for three days, Vishnu-devananda was content because they fed him dates and he was able to do his *sadhana,* Srinivasananda says. When his jailers found out who he was, they wanted to fete him and took him to a nightclub replete with smoking, drinking, and belly dancing. The only thing he approved of was the dancers' abdominal muscle control.) In 1983 the "Flying Swami" flew over the Berlin Wall to show that "only man-made boundaries separate East from West, nation from nation, man from man."

The intensity of Swami Vishnu's mission was matched by his personality. "People had told me how terrible Swami Vishnu was," Srinivasananda recalls. "He didn't have time for any nonsense, and some people could not deal with that." But from the moment he met Swami Vishnu, the fit was perfect. "Swamiji taught people to swim by throwing them in, and that was my way of learning anyway, so there was a close connection." Within three months Srinivasananda was teaching classes at the ashram. The following summer he took both the basic and advanced teacher training courses, and five months after that he was ordained as a monk in the Order of Sannyasa.

Then as now, the daily Sivananda ashram schedule begins with meditation and chanting

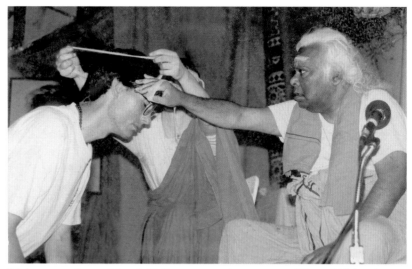

Srinivasananda receiving initiation as an acharya, *one of Swami Vishnu's senior disciples and teachers, in 1989.*

from six a.m. to eight a.m., followed by two hours of asana and *pranayama*—all before breakfast. The ensuing day of service and study ends with another two-hour asana practice, dinner, and a program of chanting, meditation, and talks on yoga philosophy and scriptures. Although the approach focuses on postures and breath work, "in the back of all Swamiji's teachings was the vision of Advaita Vedanta, the nondualistic underpinnings of yoga philosophy, of the unity of all existence," Srinivasananda says. "Swami Sivananda had always said that if you can't put Vedanta into practice, it's a waste of time. That was Swamiji's approach too."

During that first winter, when temperatures fell to forty below zero, Srinivasananda worked outside in the forest maintaining cross-country ski trails and also helped edit Vishnu-devananda's second book, *Meditation and Mantras,* a discourse on the practical applications of Yoga and Vedanta. Srinivasananda learned the Hindu chanting and song so vital to the Sivananda practice. He even taught a few classes in French. "So I got everything I was looking for, the entire list," he says.

Then, in September 1978, Srinivasananda was nudged out of the nest. Resident teachers in the Sivananda organization are cyclically assigned to centers of which there are now twenty-five worldwide. Srinivasananda served first in Chicago, then at the Woodbourne, New York, ashram he now directs, and then in Paris, where he was sent to head up a center for the first time. "That was another sink-or-swim situation," he says. "My French was not very good, so I did a two-month intensive at the Alliance Française." Just at that time, when Srinivasananda faced these challenges and a period of indecision about whether to continue as a swami, Vishnu-devananda went into seclusion somewhere in India and could not be consulted.

Back in Val Morin, students would go to see Swami Vishnu with their problems. "He would say, 'Write them down, and we'll discuss what to do afterward—but when you write, make sure it's only on one page,'" Srinivasananda recalls. "He made sure people were concise and that they did not get lost in emotion. He considered these problems a mere question of vibration—which from my experience is a deep truth. If you're in a negative place and practice asanas or *pranayama,* or mantra meditation, the problem is often completely transformed. You can deal with it from a place of being centered and strong and relaxed. So Swami Vishnu would say, 'What you need to do is more *japa* [repetition of mantra].' Although he usually

Practicing Shining Skull Breath Expansion (*Kapalabhati Pranayama*)

1. Choose a comfortable cross-legged position that allows you to sit tall, with your shoulders over your hips and the back of your head in line with your back. Swami Srinivasananda, shown in Adept's pose (*Siddhasana*), recommends elevating your seat as necessary ❶ to ensure that you do not collapse through the shoulders and chest. Begin sharp, pumping exhalations through the nostrils again and again. The exhalations are quick and strong, while the inhalations are relaxed. Here you exaggerate the natural movement that your diaphragm (the dome-shaped muscular partition that separates the chest and abdominal cavity) makes all day long if you breathe properly. When you inhale, the diaphragm drops down and the intercostal muscles between the ribs expand as the lungs fill. When you exhale, the diaphragm retracts, pushing air out of the lungs. By sharply pumping the diaphragm, we not only heighten its function and efficacy, we also increase the capacity of our lungs to empty and fill. A Sivananda asana class generally begins with three to five rounds of fifty to one hundred pumpings of *Kapalabhati*.

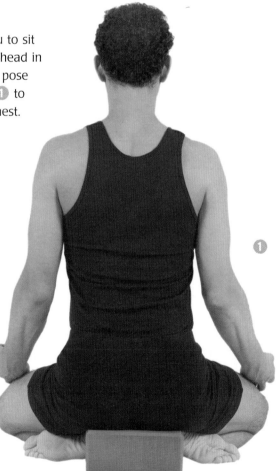

wouldn't discuss the problem directly, during a lecture on Vedanta or yoga, you could feel that he would be talking specifically to you. It was an incredible art."

In 1982 Srinivasananda renounced his monastic vows to marry a fellow practitioner he had met in France. Swami Vishnu initially withheld his blessing but changed his mind and instructed the couple to "practice and teach and become an example of how powerful householders can be in spiritual life." For the next twenty-one years they lived, worked, and raised a child within the community. "I would say that along with my experience with Swami Vishnu, my relationship with my wife, the way we matured together spiritually and emotionally, was the greatest teaching I have had," Srinivasananda says. But in March 2003 he chose to renew his vows, driven by a visitation in a dream—this time from someone who called him to stand up and commit one hundred percent to his yoga path by reconfirming his *sannyasin* vows.

"The main vow you take as a swami is that you will not have fear of anything in this world, and that you will not give fear to anyone in this world," Srinivasananda explains. "My decision to retake Sannyasa was to affirm that yes, I'm committed to peace." Srinivasananda's wife, also a senior Sivananda Yoga teacher, shares that perspective and is studying to become a Buddhist nun with Thich Nhat Hanh. Srinivasananda continues to direct the Sivananda Yoga Ranch in Woodbourne, New York, and trains yoga teachers internationally. He is also the editor of the organization's magazine, *Yoga Life,* through which he, like Vishnu-devananda, works to awaken people to the possibility of peace through *ahimsa* and personal transformation.

On the first anniversary of the terrorist bombings of September 11, 2001, Srinivasananda released an issue featuring articles by Thich Nhat Hanh, John Robbins, and Noam Chomsky, as well as his own account of teaching in Iran six months after the attacks. "What I was trying to do in the magazine was to show the spectrum of people standing up for truth, understanding, and peace. If you kill all the possible terrorists in the world, by the time you're finished, there's not going to be anybody left. Our country has this policy now—which is not to condemn America but to say we're in a time of incredible possibilities for transformation. If we don't transform toward unity and peace, we'll destroy the planet. But if we are able to transform our attitude, we have the knowledge, technology, organization, and communication to create any sort of paradise."

In Srinivasananda's eyes, ashram life plays an important role in that effort and in the progression of yoga in America. "Outwardly, the teaching stays the same," he says. "But the evolution is taking place in the individuals who are practicing. Swami Sivananda and Swami Vishnu touched millions of people with their dedication to and understanding of yoga, and the teaching remains alive and vibrant through those of us who carry it on now. It's not by innovations that we evolve, but by going deeper into the practice."

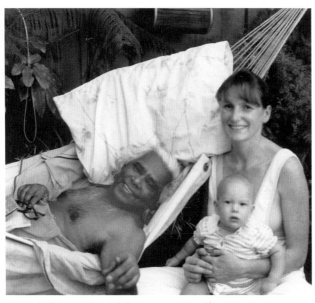

Swami Vishnu with Srinivasananda's wife, Laksmi, and daughter, Sivakami, at the Sivananda center in Los Angeles in 1984.

2. In the Sivananda tradition *Kapalabhati* is generally taught in combination with Alternate Nostril Breathing *(Anuloma Viloma Pranayama)* 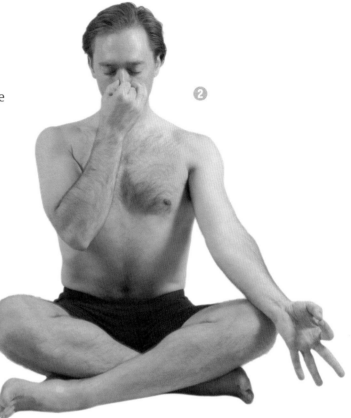, at the beginning of the class. *Anuloma Viloma* is said to bring the left and right hemispheres of the brain into sync. Arrange your left hand into *chin* or *jnana mudra,* by tucking the tip of your forefinger into the pad of the thumb. Bend the first two fingers of your right hand toward the palm in *vishnu mudra.* Alternately, use your right thumb to block off your right nostril and your right ring finger and pinky to close off your left nostril. To begin the practice, exhale through both nostrils, then block off the right nostril as you inhale through the left for four seconds. Block off both nostrils and retain the breath for sixteen seconds. Then exhale through the right nostril for eight seconds. Inhale through the right nostril for four seconds, then block off both nostrils and retain for sixteen seconds. Then release your right ring finger and pinky and exhale through the left for eight seconds. Do three rounds like this, eventually building up to twenty rounds.

Pranayama should be done on an empty stomach and is traditionally practiced after asana. But *Kapalabhati*—considered both a *kriya,* or cleansing practice, and a *pranayama*—is used to start classes in many styles, probably due to the wide influence of Sivananda Yoga training.

3. *Kumbhaka,* or retention, is standard in *pranayama* practice. Sivananda classes encourage forty-five- to sixty- to ninety-second breath retention between rounds of *Kapalabhati.* But the *bandhas,* or locks (p. 29), so freely recommended in most American yoga classes today are not taught to beginners in a Sivananda asana class. "Swami Vishnu's instructions were that people should practice *Anuloma Viloma* for six months before starting to practice *bandhas,*" Swami Srinivasananda says. "In our tradition we teach the *bandhas* separately from *pranayama* to make sure students understand and have control over them before they start using them."

Krishna Das
Devotional Chanting
(Kirtan)

When Krishna Das sings, the sound is so purely beautiful that you want to smile, weep, and join in all at once. But he insists that none of it has anything to do with him.

KD, as his fans call him, first heard of the enigmatic Indian saint called Neem Karoli Baba, or Maharaj-ji, thirty-three years ago. From that moment on he gave himself over to the adoration of the divine presence he says he is blessed to have known. But his devotion is so great that if Maharaj-ji did not exist, it would have been necessary for KD to invent him.

When KD was seventeen, a friend gave him a copy of Paramahansa Yogananda's *Autobiography of a Yogi.* "I was mind-blown by the book, and I believed everything in there," he says. "It was almost like I remembered it all, it seemed so right." More than the eyebrow-raising miracles related in the story, KD identified with the concept of *bhakti* yoga, the path of devotion that bound Yogananda to his fate of Self-discovery. KD had recognized the predominance of that aspect of his own personality during a couple of experiences with the natural hallucinogen peyote, given to him by the friend who had lent him the book. The illumination faded as the drug wore off, though, leaving him feeling empty and sad.

In 1965, when KD finished high school, he went to California and spent a week at the Self Realization Fellowship in Encinitas, the beautiful cliffside center that was so meaningful for Erich Schiffmann. The visit held little magic for KD, though. "The residents were extremely conservative and renunciation-oriented, and I was a crazed guitar-playing hippie, so I just didn't feel a connection." KD had been awarded a basketball scholarship to Brandeis University that was rescinded due to a leg injury in his senior year. So he was

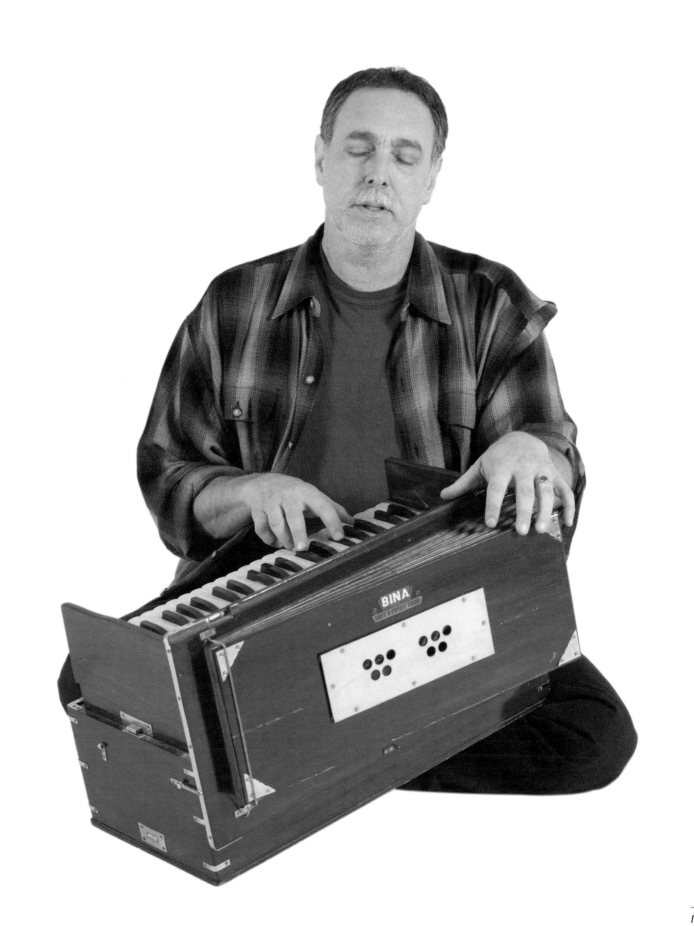

THE YOGA OF THE PRACTICE: "Why do people feel good chanting? Who knows. I could come up with some version of why, but the bottom line is that we're beginning to turn toward that place in ourselves where our essence lives, toward that place where we are happiness and we are love. Everybody knows what that place is. At the same time we're letting go of external, superficial identities and attachments. When you begin to let go of the mind and all the suffering it causes, you get happy—even if it's just for a moment and you don't know why."

HOW DO STUDENTS MISS IT? "Mostly because they think it's a musical experience instead of an expression of the longing for love. People are searching all the time for the things they think are going to give them that, but the love is already within us; it's just covered over. It's like we have some very dirty sunglasses on, so we can't see clearly where we're aiming. We keep grabbing the wrong things. Singing is the practice of developing better aim.

"It's also a question of how much people are in touch with their own pain. You already tried sex, drugs, and rock 'n' roll, none of which did what they promised to do for any length of time. You've already made the money and lost it, or made the money but now you're sitting alone in a big empty house totally unhappy, or you're surrounded by family who bring you a certain amount of happiness but not the kind of happiness you long for. People won't do practice unless they recognize that they're hurting. It's a question of how much truth you can bear and how good your aim is."

HOW TO MAKE SURE YOU CONNECT: "By understanding that chanting is meditation, a spiritual practice. It's not about whether you can carry a tune or keep a beat. You also need to realize that nobody is listening to you. It's about overcoming the shyness at first—opening up a little bit and relaxing."

"As the mind gets quieter, you begin to enter into blissful states of consciousness that also pass. But your true self never comes or goes. It is uncontrived, uncreated. It is who you are, and you learn how to reside in that. Chanting is part of paving the way for grace."

ready to "go be a lumberjack with the guy who gave me the peyote and *Autobiography of a Yogi*" when he got a call from the basketball coach at Stonybrook University on Long Island. He accepted the coach's offer to play basketball there.

It was an unhappy experience, exacerbated by drug use and unrelieved even by the relative success of the band he was playing in. Throughout it all KD continued to delve into the contemplative traditions "in my own way," he says. "You've got to remember, there wasn't a yoga studio on every block." He went to New York City to attend talks by Swami Satchidananda—"he was very beautiful, but there was no heart connection there, either"—and he met Swami Chidananda when the master visited Ananda Ashram in Monroe, New York. But nothing touched KD like the experience he had upon meeting his guru, in the person of the American yoga pioneer Ram Dass.

In the winter of 1968 Ram Dass, newly back from his travels in India, was holding court on the lawn of his father's estate in New Hampshire, where a campground's worth of hippies had flocked to be near the counterculture pioneer. Ram Dass, in his previous incarnation as Richard Alpert, had taught psychology at Harvard until he was thrown out in 1963 for his overzealous experimentation with psilocybin, which helped initiate the psychedelic revolution. When he journeyed to India four years later, he fell in league with a twenty-three-old American named Bhagavan Das, who had been wandering the continent for five years in nothing but a dhoti, the traditional garb of holy men. Bhagavan Das spoke fluent Hindi but spent most of his time singing the chants he had learned in his travels and honed to perfection at the feet of Neem Karoli Baba, his guru, whom he took Ram Dass to see.

Lore has it that Neem Karoli Baba spared a shopkeeper's life by forewarning him of his impending murder. It is also said he regularly fed huge gatherings of people on one portion of food. What Ram Dass perceived when he met him surpassed all legend: Maharaj-ji could not only read his mind, but seemed to love him regardless. The quality of that love, and of the man's essence, felt like God to him, just as it did to the thousands of Indian disciples who had been following him for decades. The experience shook Ram Dass to the core. The reverberations were still palpable in New Hampshire.

"The instant I sat down with Ram Dass, I realized that all the things I was longing for in my heart were real, and not a dream," KD says. "And that was the development of faith." For the next year and a half KD insisted that he wanted to be with Maharaj-ji. But as Ram Dass explained in his 1971 book, *Be Here Now,* which joined the canon of spiritual literature for an entire generation of Americans, he had been forbidden to divulge his guru's name or whereabouts. Eventually, KD cajoled him into providing the address of a devotee in India, who let KD know when and where to show up. And so he did, along with two fellow seekers. (One was Daniel Goleman, who now defines American spirituality by reforming it into lectures and books on developmental and corporate psychology.)

KD describes his experiences at Neem Karoli Baba's temple in September 1970 by saying that being there "was better than anything I had ever felt. We didn't meditate or do asana. We just tried to be with Maharaj-ji as much as possible. We sang for him because we found out he liked it. It was a way to bribe him to spend time with us."

> *"The* sankirtans *or musical gatherings are an effective form of yoga or spiritual discipline, necessitating intense concentration, absorption in the seed thought and sound. Because man himself is an expression of the Creative Word, sound exercises on him a potent and immediate effect. Great religious music of East and West bestows joy on man because it causes a temporary vibratory awakening of one of his occult spinal centers* [chakras]. *In those blissful moments a dim memory comes to him of his divine origin."*
> —Paramahansa Yogananda
> *Autobiography of a Yogi*

Like the Hindu deity Krishna, Neem Karoli Baba would hide, then appear, then hide again, KD says. "If he ran away for all or part of the winter, as he usually did, we would go do meditation courses in Bodh Gaya"—the site of the Buddha's enlightenment—"or whatever we could to fill the time till Maharaj-ji showed up again. He would leave one place and show up somewhere else. We'd all go there and hang out and then he'd leave and show up in another place. It was wild. You only found him if he wanted you to find him."

More and more Westerners began turning up at the temple. "By spring there were twenty or thirty hanging around, but you could only stay if Maharaj-ji let you," KD says. He let KD stay a long time, but one day in March 1973, the guru looked up, saw him, and said, "You go back to America; you have attachment there." And KD knew it to be true.

"My heart was constricted in its own way, and my understanding of things was very simplistic. I still had lots of desires and attachments I needed to work through." He returned to the U.S. and spent the next six months mostly thinking about when he might return to his guru. But on September 11, 1973, Neem Karoli Baba left his body to enter *mahasamadhi,* as yogis phrase it. For KD, the loss was incalculable.

"I had felt that I was in the presence of God,"

he says, "and all I wanted was to be in that presence. No matter what I heard or read about how God is in everybody, the emotional reality was that I was attached to being with him physically, so when he wasn't there I sank like a stone for a long time. That itself became the path: to find my way back to his presence."

Asanas were little help. "I do asana when my body gets

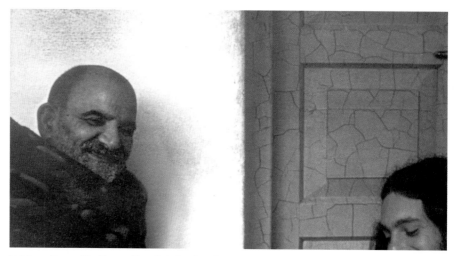

Krishna Das with Neem Karoli Baba in 1971.

stiff and I need a crane to get out of bed in the morning, but asana has never been part of my spiritual work," KD says. "Doing good, being good, sitting this way, breathing this way—it may get you high, but it does not necessarily make you fall in love. And ultimately we're trying to fall in love with ourselves. Practice can help clean the mirror of the heart, where once you see your own beauty you fall in love. But somebody like Maharaj-ji reflects that beauty because he is that beauty. He has become the presence that lives within all hearts, and so he does it for everyone and anyone who is ready or whom he chooses." KD was ready or chosen again in 1984, when while visiting a temple on a trip to India, he felt his guru return to him. "I saw that I hadn't lost him, that in fact he'd been with me all the time but I would not allow myself to feel him because I was so angry that he had died."

The experience nudged him to play out a bit instead of just chanting with the folks who knew him as "Maharaj-ji's *kirtan* guy," he says. "When you're sitting with people who don't know what chanting is about, you have to really be present. You have to really do the practice. I saw that there were places in my own heart I would never access if I didn't force myself to do that." And so he did.

KD's *kirtans* seem like rock concerts minus the smoke. His highly popular recordings have made him something of a cult figure among nouveau hippies and dyed-in-the-wool yogis alike.

"It's not that big a deal," he says. "I can go to a supermarket without the cashiers blushing. And I don't gauge the success of the chanting on how many people come; I gauge it on how I feel on a daily basis, which is also getting better."

If you laugh and cry and sing during *kirtan* with KD, it's all good. "Emotions come up, and chanting uses the energy of emotions. But it's all channeled into the Name"—the practice of repeating these names for God that have been sung for millennia. Krishna Das's own name was originally Jeff Kagel, which he still uses when he orders anything online, he says. The names Neem Karoli Baba gave his disciples—Krishna Das means "servant of God"—come from the line of Hanuman, the Hindu monkey god who leapt across the ocean in the name of divine love. "We aspire to that kind of presence; we want to be that way in the world—serving God in every being," KD says. "It's gratifying to know that my guru is using me to touch people. I show up and sing. But Maharaj-ji opens people's hearts." When you listen to Krishna Das, you hear what he means.

Caught in the storm,
battered by waves,
the ship of my life
was blown off course
By the winds of desire.

My breath rises in me,
The breath of the heart.
The sweet breath.
The sacred breath leads me in.

The winds begin to die down
and the waters calm.
I have found a haven for my heart,
In the Harbor of the Name.

—Krishna Das

Vyaas Houston
Speaking Yoga

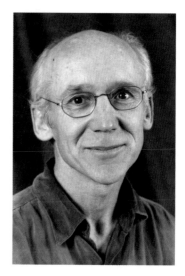

Although he does asanas every day, Vyaas Houston's primary practice for the past thirty-one years has been the language that has kept yoga's teachings alive. "Knowledge of Sanskrit," he says, "lets you grasp the subtleties of yoga."

Like most practitioners, Vyaas first heard Sanskrit in an invocational mantra chanted at the beginning of an asana class. For him the resonance was particularly enduring. "Chanting is beautiful whether you're pronouncing the Sanskrit correctly or not," he says. "But once you start pronouncing it properly, you get so much more enjoyment out of it. And when you know the meaning of what you are chanting, there's a steady, direct penetration that takes you ever deeper."

Back in 1968 Vyaas, or Tuck, as he was then called, was worried about the draft and was having a hard time in his undergraduate studies at Syracuse University. While taking summer school classes in sociology and calculus to maintain his academic standing, he ran into a friend who had taken up yoga and was extolling its virtues. Vyaas picked up a copy of *The Complete Illustrated Book of Yoga,* by Swami Vishnu-devananda, and "immediately took to it," he says. "I was just amazed at the changes." He started a daily practice of asana, meditation, and concentration exercises and found that the practice helped him ace his courses with little or no study. He kept it up when the fall semester resumed.

After graduation Vyaas spent a winter living "Thoreau-style" in the woods. He then began to teach hatha yoga, picking up a certificate through the Integral Yoga Institute along the way. As his friends increasingly became people involved in yoga, he heard about Ananda Ashram in Monroe, New York. The ashram had been established seven

THE SANSKRIT ALPHABET

संस्कृतवर्णमाला SAŃSKṚTA-VARṆA-MĀLĀ

vowels *(svara)*

simple — short & long:

अ A	आ Ā	इ I	ई Ī	उ U	ऊ Ū		ऋ Ṛ	ॠ R̄
guttural		*palatal*		*labial*			*cerebral*	

diphthongs — long:

				anusvāra	*visarga*		
ए E	ऐ AI	ओ O	औ AU	अं AṀ	अः AḤ	ऌ Ḷ	ॡ L̄
							dental

consonants *(vyañjana)*

mutes *(sparsha)*

class - location	hard (voiceless)		soft (voiced)		
	simple	aspirate	simple	aspirate	nasal
gutturals - throat	क KA	ख KHA	ग GA	घ GHA	ङ ṄA
palatals - middle of mouth	च CA (cha)	छ CHA (chha)	ज JA	झ JHA	ञ ÑA
cerebrals - roof of mouth	ट ṬA	ठ ṬHA	ड ḌA	ढ ḌHA	ण ṆA
dentals - teeth	त TA	थ THA	द DA	ध DHA	न NA
labials - lips	प PA	फ PHA	ब BA	भ BHA	म MA

semi-vowels *(antastha)* — soft

य YA	र RA	ल LA	व VA
palatal	*cerebral*	*dental*	*labial*

sibilants — hard & pure aspirate — soft *(ūshman)*

श ṢA (sha)	ष ṢA (sha)	स SA	ह HA
palatal	*cerebral*	*dental*	*guttural*

special compound consonants: क्ष KṢA   त्र TRA   ज्ञ JÑA (gña)

years earlier by Sri Brahmananda Sarasvati, or Dr. Mishra as he was called then. Vyaas had picked up Brahmananda's *Textbook of Yoga Psychology,* a modern treatise on the *Yoga Sutras,* "but I didn't begin to comprehend it and just put it down," he says. On a friend's recommendation he went to see Dr. Mishra anyway, and in doing so, found his guru and his calling.

In 1971 Sri Brahmananda was teaching Sanskrit at Ananda Ashram all day every day. When Vyaas entered the large white house where residents lived and studied, he was greeted by a roomful of people chanting responsively. He sat down, joined in, and was instantly carried away by the beauty of the language and by Sri Brahmananda's passion for it. "When he chanted, every atom of his body seemed to dissolve into a state of vibration," he says. "By duplicating his sounds, we all miraculously went along for the ride."

Vyaas accompanied his guru to San Francisco, where Sri Brahmananda Sarasvati taught at the California Institute of Asian Studies and opened a

---

LOKA SAMASTHA SUKHINO BHAVANTU

लोकाः समस्ताः सुखिनो भवन्तु

"May all beings in the world be happy," is the translation of this ancient chant commonly heard in yoga classes today. If its sentiment sounds saccharine, ask whether you don't wish this for yourself. See what it takes to wish it for everybody else, and discover the power of understanding the language of yoga.

---

second center in 1972. Vyaas taught yoga in the area and combined those earnings with his life's savings to tour the world with his teacher. "It was wonderful to see the energy he had when he spoke in Hindi, his native tongue," he notes.

"Vyaas," the spiritual name Brahmananda gave him, literally translates as "the diameter of a circle." But it is more widely associated with the near-mythic sage said to have written the *Mahabarata,* which contains the *Bhagavad Gita,* the bedrock of Hinduism. Since this seer is also credited with having organized the Vedas—the oldest literature known to mankind—the name has come to mean 'one who arranges.' Vyaas did exactly that when he returned to the Ananda Ashram as program director. From 1975 through 1983 he organized weekend workshops and conferences at the ashram, while earning a master's degree in Sanskrit at Columbia University in New York City.

"When I started out, I was really absorbed in hatha yoga," Vyaas says. "But when Sanskrit came along, hatha became secondary. Chanting the language turns your body into a cosmic resonator. As hatha yoga prepares the body to sit for meditation, through mantras and sacred teachings, Sanskrit provides clarity and guidance toward stillness of mind, peace, and Self-knowledge. The entire tradition ultimately comes down to sound."

In the *Yoga Sutras,* Patanjali describes *Isvara pranidhana*—devotion to *Isvara,* a concept of the

---

"We normally associate mantra with some meaningless sound we repeat mechanically until we are put in some kind of trance. Actually, mantra is quite different than this. Just as yoga practice requires a special power or *shakti* for it to be effective, for mantra to work there must be a conscious creative energization of sound and meaning. The more deeply we can inquire into things, the more our thoughts become mantra. It is something like the difference between poetry and ordinary speech. Mantra must have at least as much creative empowerment as a good poem. Without this creative vision, mantra may be no more than a form of self-hypnosis."

—David Frawley,
Sanskrit, the Language of the Vedas

THE SOUND OF THE UNIVERSE

"All Mantras are hidden in Om, which is the abstract, highest Mantra of the cosmos. Correctly pronounced the sound proceeds from the navel, with a deep and harmonious vibration, and gradually manifests itself at the upper part of the nostrils. The larynx and palate are the sounding boards; no part of the tongue or palate is touched. 'AH' is the first sound the vocal apparatus can utter; M is the last. As the U is pronounced in between the sound rolls from the root of the tongue to the end of the sounding board of the mouth, where M is produced by closing the lips.

Pronounced merely as spelled, Om will have a certain effect upon the nervous system, and will benefit the psyche. Pronounced correctly, it arouses and transforms every atom in the physical body, setting up new vibrations and awakening dormant physical and mental powers."

—Swami Vishnu-devananda, *Meditation and Mantras*

Om, said to contain all the sounds of the universe, is omnipresent and audible before and after you make it. You can hear it in the air conditioner, in your heart, in a car alarm, if you listen well and deeply enough. The description of Om in the *Yoga Sutras* is *pranava*—that which is ever new. "Om is ever new in the sense of listening in deep meditation to the inner sound, which can be reached by chanting it," Vyaas Houston says. "At a finer, subtler level, Om is the sound of creation where creation is one resonance. And the method by which one's *citta*, or consciousness, expands into that is by listening."

Swami Sivananda, who like Dr. Mishra was a physician before he became a yogi, said that the vibrations produced by the continuous chanting of Om stimulate the activity of the pituitary and pineal glands through a massage-like action in the nasal cavity. "Vibrations directed at locations in the palate definitely affect your brain," Vyaas says. "So when you chant Om and you're sensitive to that, it's like taking this wave and neutralizing everything to create a sense of total peace."

The beauty of yoga is that its efficacy is absolutely empirical—which goes for everything from asanas to *pranayama* to meditation to the practice of chanting. Place your hand on the top of your head and feel the top of your skull vibrate your palm as you repeatedly make the sound mmm. Remember that the roof of your nasal cavity forms the floor of your brain. Then forget all that, rest your hand back down on your thigh, and "submerge yourself in the ocean of pulsation," as Sri Brahmananda Sarasvati told his students. "Feel the pulsation of energy from your body to the entire universe, the sun, moon, and stars, and from the entire universe back to you." "Om is the very first name," Krishna Das says. "It's the name of the whole."

Lord not necessarily akin to the Judeo-Christian paradigm—as a practice of sound. "The sutra *Tasya vacakah pranavah* declares that the expression of *Isvara* is the *pranava,* the name of Om," Vyaas says. Sound, specifically recitation of texts, is equally central to Patanjali's definition of *Svadhyaya,* or Self-study—another of the delineated steps on the path to attaining yoga and one that has had tremendous effect for Vyaas.

"Sanskrit for me has been a tool for penetrating deeper into the teachings and into meditation," he says. For millennia, teachings like the *Sutras* were handed down orally, "so you get this feeling of being connected. When it comes to reading the Vedas, the language is so crystal clear, it's as if you are there. That was the gift of these great writers and poets of ancient times: to create images of consciousness through literature, philosophy, stories, and myths that reveal the beauty of Sanskrit as a means for doing that. Reading the literature in its original language brings you directly to their vision. It's a maturing process that obviously takes time."

In 1988 Vyaas left Ananda Ashram, where he eventually served as president, to start up the American Sanskrit Institute, now based in Warwick, New York. Because dropout rates from Sanskrit courses are high at the universities that offer them, Vyaas thought carefully about how it could best be taught. Using yogically evolved theories regarding success, failure, and stick-to-itiveness, he insists he can teach anyone the mathematically precise language and strongly recommends its study for any serious practitioner of yoga.

"It's one of the most empowering tools there is," he says. "I never would have understood the teachings to the degree I have if I hadn't been looking at them in the original language. Sanskrit, through its sound and its specialized vocabulary, just does not translate all that well."

The man who set him on that path of discovery was the man he called his guru, a word often said to mean "remover of darkness." Vyaas, however, says it means "weighty." "When I first met Sri Brahmananda Sarasvati—and for a long time—I just wanted to be in his presence," Vyaas recalls. "He taught me an extraordinary amount. What I learned from him ultimately was not to place anyone above one's own self, that when you put someone on a pedestal, there's always an element of fear there. In the end, I had to distance myself from him in terms of my own life's course."

Vyaas remembers his guru as "a very dear friend I loved with all my heart who inspired me into the study of Sanskrit and sacred teachings and spiritual life." Yet the path was hewn the very first time Vyaas opened his mouth to chant in a hatha yoga class. "I loved the sound," he says.

ON LOVE IN SANSKRIT

The bird is in the field
as the field is in the bird.
In the grammar of Sanskrit
one can't have it
one way over the other.
Moons rise in the sky
because *Om nama sri chandra*
the adept tongue makes it so.

Guttural/palatal/dental/domal/labial
in the cosmology of Sanskrit
sound creates the round phenomenal world
our tongues are so busy talking about.
The fall of a single inflection
separates a saint from a sunset.

One has got to enunciate
in the *deva*-derived alphabet of Sanskrit
& since pronunciation's so stressed
why not admit the tip of the tongue as the *lingam*
the place all memory stores itself
where the phallic crown waits to play
in the mouth's moist *yoni* cave.

Create me create me
scores of sleeping life forms whisper
& how that tongue can whip up
quite a wonder song.
Birds? Yeah
birds fly wildly
but the field doesn't really open
until a considerable change of interest occurs.

The Tantrics say
the illusion of a separate 'I' is the veil
that keeps one's own divine nature unknown
& so the other is everything one seeks
to discover to honor
to join & become.

In the lingua of Sanskrit
mother-root of every Indo-Euro tongue
the part one plays in the art of love
is so exact.

—Kirpal Gordon

Rand Hicks
Concentration
(Dharana)

Concentration, or dharana is one of the great powers of yoga," says Rand Hicks. "Asana is *dharana* for body, and *pranayama* is *dharana* for regulation of life energy. So building the concentration from near to far in this way, we move from the body and mind toward the soul, toward the Divine in us."

When he was nineteen, Rand Hicks thought he could attain that realization by sitting alone on a mountaintop. But his spiritual quest was redefined a year later when he picked up a book called *Vivekananda: The Yogas and Other Works*. The book described one of Swami Vivekananda's early meetings with the master Sri Ramakrishna. "Vivekananda blurted out, 'Sir, you're always talking about God,'" Rand recalls. "Then he said, 'I'm a new thinker. I believe in science. Tell me: Have you seen God?' And Ramakrishna replied, 'Yes. And he's more real to me at this moment than you are.'

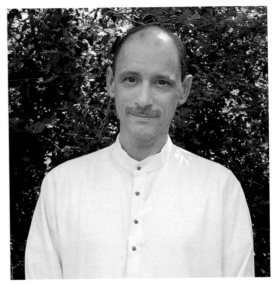

"The idea that you could have the experience of God here and now was revolutionary to me," Rand says. "After that, it was all I wanted to pursue." The route was cemented when during his university studies in philosophy and Sanskrit, he opened a book by the Indian yoga master Sri Aurobindo Ghosh. "I felt that I had read truth as well as it could be fashioned," he says. "I became deeply interested in Sri Aurobindo's work and came to see that his path was possible: that yoga is concentrated evolution in which the appreciation and affirmation of life in the world is necessary."

Sri Aurobindo Ghosh, who honed what he came to call "Integral Yoga" while jailed in 1908 for political action against Great Britain's occupation of India, always encouraged his followers to pursue the *sadhana* that suited their individual temperaments. He was as pragmatic about yoga's adaptability over time. "Yoga has long diverged from life," he said. "And the ancient systems that sought to embrace it, such as those of our Vedic forefathers, are far away from us, expressed in terms which are no longer accessible, thrown into forms which are no longer applicable. Mankind has moved forward on the current of eternal Time, and the same problem has to be approached from a new starting point."

By 1926 an ashram had grown up around Aurobindo in Pondicherry, India, "not for the renunciation of the world," he said, "but for the evolution of another kind and form of life moved by a higher spiritual consciousness." The residents of his community followed their guru's edict to bring their strong grounding in the tenets of yoga and meditation into the activities of daily life. Aurobindo's ashram has grown since those days to a thriving society of some 1000 residents and another 400 people in the International Center of Education. "There are 400 applicants for every position," Rand notes, "because they aren't charged a penny and when people finish their educational career, everybody wants to hire them. They are highly prized in the Indian economic system because they have a cultural and spiritual outlook as well as technical skills."

In June 1974, Rand flew to India to attend Benares Hindu University, which had awarded him a fellowship at the master's level to continue his study of Indian philosophy. But when he arrived, the university was closed down due to a "three-way dogfight" among the student body, which was in rebellion against the administration, and the central government, which was fighting the college administration. Classes were postponed until December, so Rand wrote to the ashram for permission to live there in the interim. He was so captivated by what he found there that he never returned to Benares.

Sri Aurobindo's teachings had long influenced masters like Swami Satchidananda, who applied the name Integral Yoga to the school of yoga he developed in the West. In 1979, Rand transplanted Aurobindo's approach to Pensacola, Florida, where he established the Integral Knowledge Study Center.

> In moments when the inner lamps are lit
> And the life's cherished guests are left outside,
> Our spirit sits alone and speaks to its gulfs.
> —Sri Aurobindo

Aurobindo's intellectual and experiential game plan, aimed toward realization of what he called Supramental Consciousness, spoke to Rand in a way that the world-denying approach of some traditions did not. "In the development of a real spiritual life, you don't need the outer trappings of the sannyasi," he says. "What you need is the inner release from attachment to forms, desires, and life powers. That is why in the *Bhagavad Gita* Krishna says again and again to Arjuna, 'Conquer and enjoy an opulent kingdom.' He doesn't say, 'Go away and become a sannyasi or a sage.' He says, 'Attain this realization in which you allow a higher consciousness and power to work through you with your full collaboration, with a heart and a mind full of Me. Take on my being and all go well. And you will enjoy.'"

Yoga turns upon three things, Rand says: concentration, purification, and surrender.

"Concentration brings purity. It's a process that has nothing to do with ethics. When you are one-pointed with the object of your attention, you become pure. After asana and *pranayama* comes *pratyahara*, withdrawal of the attention from the senses. *Pratyahara* is not an exclusionary technique by which you force out one part of your being. It is a movement that allows you to gain access to inner spaces so that you can focus your attention. Just as the breath doesn't stop while the asanas continue, in *pratyahara* you are telescoping toward your true nature. Once that inner movement begins, you are ready for dhyana, meditation."

"It is not sufficient to worship Krishna, Christ or Buddha without, if there is not the revealing and the formation of the Buddha, the Christ or Krishna in ourselves," Aurobindo wrote. In so doing, he inspired Rand Hicks and thousands of seekers to make life Divine.

Meditation
(Dhyana)

Each teacher in American Yoga might lead you differently toward the practice of seated meditation. Your own approach, like theirs, will deepen over time. After bending, twisting, and turning the body in asana practice, it is far easier to sit quietly and move beyond the fluctuations of the mind. Choose a comfortable seat with your knees at the level of your hips. Do not force yourself into some external form you cannot comfortably maintain, but instead allow your exploration of meditation to be like that of asanas—the best and truest reflection of what you are.

You can practice one-pointed concentration by following the breath, as the Buddha instructed. You can follow instead the way in which thoughts, sensations, and feelings come and go in the style of *vipassana,* which widens rather than narrows the stream of focus to train you to deconstruct the workings of the mind. As is the case with asana practice, the style that speaks to you now may not be the one you stay with all your life. "Techniques are important," Rand Hicks says. "But let us use techniques in so far as they are useful and lay them down gratefully when they are not."

Regardless of the method, the goal is the same: "The inner Guide is often veiled at first by the very intensity of our personal effort and by the ego's preoccupation with itself and its aims," Aurobindo wrote. "As we gain in clarity and the turmoil of egoistic effort gives place to calmer Self-knowledge, we recognize the source of the growing light within us. We recognize it in the essence of our being as that develops into oneness with a greater and wider existence, for we perceive that this miraculous development is not the result of our own efforts. An eternal Perfection is molding us into its own image."

One of the sweetest traditions carried on in American yoga is the simple expression of *Namaste.* "The light within me salutes the light within you," is what we say when we fold our palms together in front of our hearts.

We salute the light within us. We find it within each other. Because for all beings everywhere, now begins yoga, again and again.

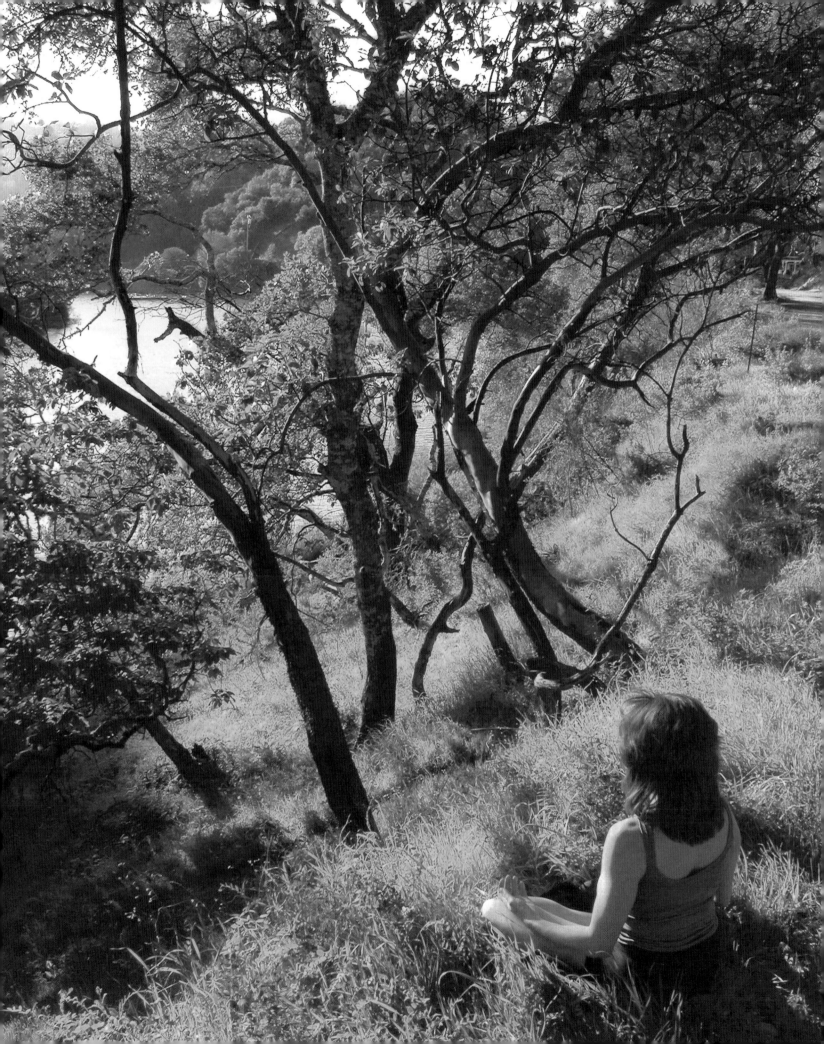

Resource List

Beryl Bender Birch

www.power-yoga.com

Books :

Power Yoga, New York,
Fireside/Simon & Schuster, 1995

Beyond Power Yoga, New York,
Fireside/Simon & Schuster, 2000

DVDs/Videos:

Power Yoga: the Practice

Power Yoga for Runners by Thom
Birch and Beryl Bender Birch

Emmy Cleaves

www.bikramyoga.com
Yoga College of India
1862 La Cienega Boulevard
Los Angeles, CA 90035
(310) 854-5800

Stephen Cope

www.kripalu.org
stephencope1@aol.com
(413) 499-3135

Books:

*Yoga and the Quest for the True
Self,* New York, Bantam, 1999

*Will Yoga and Meditation
Really Change My Life?* (ed.)
Massachusetts, Storey Publishing,
2003

The Complete Path of Yoga,
New York, Bantam, 2004

Audio Cassette/Video/CD:

Kripalu Yoga Dynamic (video)

The Yoga of Emotions,
Sounds True, 2003

Kripalu Yoga Gentle (CD)
Padma Media, 2004

Krishna Das

www.krishnadas.com

Video:

The Yoga of Chant

Audio Cassettes (music):

One Track Heart

Pilgrim Heart

Live on Earth

Breath of the Heart

Door of Faith

Audio Cassette (talk):

Pilgrim of the Heart

Nischala Joy Devi

www.abundantwellbeing.com
nd@abundantwellbeing.com
(415) 459-5336

Book:

*The Healing Path of Yoga—
Time-Honored Wisdom and
Scientifically Proven Methods
That Alleviate Stress, Open Your
Heart and Enrich Your Life,*
New York, Three Rivers Press,
2000

Audio Cassettes/CDs:

Dynamic Stillness

Relax, Move & Heal

Deep Relaxation

Sojourn to Healing

Mary Dunn

yogaoutthere.com
www.iyengarnyc.org
marydunn@earthlink.net
Iyengar Yoga Institute of New York
27 West 24th Street
Suite 800
New York, NY 10010
(212) 691-9642

Lilias Folan

www.liliasyoga.com
www.naturaljourneys.com

Books:

Lilias! Yoga Gets Better with Age

Lilias, Yoga and You

Lilias, Yoga and Your Life

David Frawley

www.vedanet.com
American Institute of
Vedic Studies
P.O. Box 8357
Santa Fe, NM 87504-8357
(505) 983-9385
Fax (505) 982-5807

Richard Freeman

www.yogaworkshop.com

Audio Cassettes/CDs/DVDs:

*The Yoga Matrix: The Body
as a Gateway to Freedom.*
(CD and cassettes)

Yoga Breathing (CD)

*Yoga with Richard Freeman:
An Introduction to Ashtanga Yoga*
(DVD/video)

*Yoga with Richard Freeman:
Ashtanga Yoga the Primary Series*
(DVD/video)

*Yoga with Richard Freeman:
Ashtanga Yoga the
Intermediate Series*
(DVD/video)

John Friend

www.anusara.com
oneyoga@anusara.com
Anusara Yoga
9400 Grogan's Mill Road,
Suite 200
The Woodlands, TX 77380
888 398-9642

Publication:
*Anusara Yoga Teacher
Training Manual*

Audio Cassette/CDs/Videos:
Yoga For Meditators (video)
*Yoga Alignment and Form:
A Home Practice Session* (video)
Anusara Yoga 101 (CD)
Anusara Yoga Essentials (CD)
*Anusara Yoga: A Weekend
Workshop* (video/audio)
*Anusara Yoga Teacher
Training* (CD)

Sharon Gannon and David Life

www.jivamuktiyoga.com
Jivamukti Yoga Center
404 Lafayette Street, 3rd Floor
New York, NY 10003

Books:
*Jivamukti Yoga: Practices
for Liberating Body and Soul*,
Gannon and Life, New York,
Ballantine Books, 2002

The Art of Yoga, Gannon and Life,
New York, Stewart, Tabori &
Chang, 2002

Cats and Dogs Are People Too,
Gannon, Jivamukti Press, 1999

Audio Cassettes/CDs/DVDs/Videos:
*Instructional Class (*audio CDs)
Instructional Class (visual DVDs)
Meditation (CD)
Neti-Neti Audio Letter Remix (CD)
What Is Yoga (video)
Asana Dance (video)

Rand Hicks

randhicks@aol.com
Integral Knowledge Study Center
221 Clematis Street
Pensacola, FL 32503
(850) 433-3435

Vyaas Houston

www. americansanskrit.com
sanskrit@sbcglobal.net
American Sanskrit Institute
Six Main Street
Chester, CT 06412

Krishna Kaur

krishna108@attbi.com
(323) 938-8397

Your Own Greatness Affirmed
(Y.O.G.A.) Inc. sponsors:
"Yoga for Youth"
1035 South Cloverdale Avenue
Los Angeles, CA 90019
(323) 735-0500
www.yogaforyouth.org
whatsup@yogaforyouth.org

International Association of
Black Yoga Teachers (IABYT)
P.O. Box 360922
Los Angeles, CA 90036
(213) 833-6371
www.blackyogateachers.com
yoga@blackyogateachers.com

Gary Kraftsow

www.viniyoga.com
info@viniyoga.com
For information about Gary
Kraftsow's American Viniyoga
Institute Teacher-Therapist
Training Programs, as well as
retreats, workshops, and
educational products, contact:
American Viniyoga Institute
P.O. Box 88
Makawao, HI 96768
(808) 572-1414

Books:
*Yoga for Wellness:
Healing with the Timeless
Teachings of Viniyoga*,
New York, Penguin, 1999

*Yoga for Transformation:
Ancient Teachings and Practices
for Healing the Body, Mind, and
Heart*, New York, Penguin, 2002

Audio Cassette:
Yoga for Wellness

Judith Hanson Lasater

www.judithlasater.com
judithyoga@aol.com
(415) 759-7439

Books:
*30 Essential Yoga Poses:
For Beginning Students and
Their Teachers*, Berkeley, CA:
Rodmell Press, 2003

Living Your Yoga: Finding the Spiritual in Everyday Life, Berkeley, CA: Rodmell Press, 2000

Relax and Renew: Restful Yoga for Stressful Times, Berkeley, CA: Rodmell Press, 1995

Richard Miller

www.nondual.com
rmiller@nondual.com
Explorations in Stillness
Anahata Publications
P.O. Box 1673
Sebastopol, CA 95473
(707) 823-5023

Books:

"Welcoming All That Is: Nonduality, Yoga Nidra and the Play of Opposites in Psychotherapy," in Prendergast, J., Fenner, P., Crystal, P. (eds.), *The Sacred Mirror, Nondualism and Psychotherapy,* MN: Paragon House, 2003

"The Search for Oneness," in Cope, Stephen (ed.), *Will Yoga and Meditation Really Change My Life?* Massachusetts, Storey Publishing, 2003

Articles and Audio Cassettes available through Anahata Publications:

Infinite Awakening Workbook for Learning the Practice of Yoga Nidra Meditation

Breathing for Life: The Art of and Science of the Breath

Longing for Liberation and the Yoga Sutra of Patañjali

Mudra: *Gateways to Self-Understanding* (article and workbook)

Healing Sciatica: The Therapeutic Application of Yoga on Sciatica Audio Cassettes:
Infinite Awakening: Yoga Nidra Meditation

Breathing for Life

Non-Dual Meditation

Pranayama, *The Breath of Life*

Yoga Sutra *of Patañjali*

Tim Miller

www.ashtangayogacenter.com
Ashtanga Yoga Center
118 West E Street
Encinitas, CA 92024
(760) 632-7093

Dharma Mittra

www.dharmayogacenter.com
www.yogaasanaposter.com
Dharma Yoga Center
297 Third Avenue
New York, NY 10010
(212) 889-8160 or
(212) 253-1289

Dharma Yoga Catskill
Retreat Center
P.O. Box 734
Roscoe, NY 12776
(607) 498-5507

Shir Dharma Mittra's Teacher Training Certification programs for 200 hours and 500 hours, held yearly
(Yoga Alliance affiliated).
(212) 253-1289

Publications:

Master Yoga Chart of 908 Postures, Dharma Mittra, 1984
www.yogaasanaposter.com
(212) 253-1289

Yoga Course Chart for Beginner & Intermediate Levels, Dharma Mittra, 1975
(212) 253-1289

Asanas, 608 Yoga Poses, Novato, CA: New World Library, 2003
(415) 884-2100

John Robbins

www.foodrevolution.org

Books:

The Food Revolution: How Your Diet Can Help Save Your Life and Our World, with Dean Ornish M.D., Conari Press, 2001

Diet for a New America, H. J. Kramer, 1998

Erich Schiffmann

www.movingintostillness.com

Books:

Yoga: The Spirit and Practice of Moving into Stillness, New York, Simon & Schuster, 1996

The Joy of Yoga, contributor

Videos:

Yoga Mind & Body with Ali MacGraw

Beginning Yoga

Yoga Inversions

Live 1

Live 2

Swami Srinivasananda

www.sivananda.org
swamisrinivasan@sivananda.org

Articles written and edited for the *Sivananda YogaLife* Magazine
www.sivananda.org/publications/

Edited:

The Complete Illustrated Book of Yoga

Meditation and Mantras

Sivananda Upanishads
(all by the
Swami Vishnu-devananda)

Sivananda Video Guide to Yoga

Sivananda Yoga Teachers Training Manual
(all by the Sivananda Yoga Vedanta Center)

Lighting the Lamp of Wisdom A Week Inside a Yoga Ashram,
Skylight Paths (by John Ittner)

Books by the Sivananda Yoga Center:

The Sivananda Companion to Yoga

DK Living: Yoga Mind & Body,
Dorling Kindersley, 1998

Learn Yoga in a Weekend

The Yoga Cookbook: Vegetarian Food for Body & Mind

Hatha Yoga Pradipika
with commentary by
Swami Vishnu-devananda

Patricia Sullivan

www.yogazen.com

Patricia Walden

Book:

The Woman's Book of Yoga and Health, with Linda Sparrowe,
Shambhala Publications 2002

Videos:

Yoga for Beginners

Yoga for Beginners 2

PM Practice for Beginners

Yoga for Flexibility

Rodney Yee

www.yeeyoga.com
www.piedmontyoga.com
(Rodney's yoga studio) or
Piedmont Yoga Studio
(510) 652-3336
To purchase products:
www.gaiam.com or
800 869-3446

Book:

Yoga: The Poetry of the Body,
New York, St. Martin's Press,
2002

Audio Cassettes/CDs/DVDs/Videos:

Yoga for Strength (video, 1992)

Yoga for Relaxation (video, 1992;
DVD, 2000)

Yoga for Energy (video, 1995)

Yoga for Meditation
(video, 1996; DVD, 2000)

AM Yoga
(video, 1998; DVD, 1999)

Yoga Remedies for Natural Healing (video, 1998)

Yoga for Abs
(video, 1998; DVD, 1999)

Yoga for Back Care (video, 1998)

Power Yoga for Stamina
(video, 1999; DVD, 2000)

Power Yoga for Strength
(video, 1999; DVD, 2000)

Yoga for Two (video, 1999)

The Art of Breath & Relaxation
(video, 1999)

Power Yoga for Flexibility
(video, 1999; DVD, 2000)

Yoga for the Upper Body
(video & DVD, 1999)

Yoga Conditioning for Athletes
(video, 2000)

Yoga for Intermediates
(video, 2000)

Back Care for Beginners
(video, 2001)

Yoga Conditioning for Life
(video, 2002)

Power Yoga for Beginners
(video, 2003)

The Art of Breath & Relaxation
(audio, 1997)

Yoga Break (CD, 1999)

Family Yoga (video, 2003)

Women's posture models' clothing courtesy of
The Marika Group, Inc.
www.marika.com

Props provided courtesy of
Hugger-Mugger
Yoga Products
www.huggermugger.com

Index Page numbers in **bold** refer to illustrations and captions.

Yoga Citations

Page 9: *Sri Swami Satchidananda: Apostle of Peace* by Sita Bardow (Integral Yoga Distribution, 1986)
Page 18: *Light on Yoga* by B.K.S. Iyengar (Schocken Books; Revised edition, January 1995) p. 44
Page 31: "Passage to India" from *Leaves of Grass* by Walt Whitman (Barnes & Noble Classics Edition, 1993) pp. 342–350
Page 93: *The Heart of Yoga* by T.K.V. Desikachar (Inner Traditions International Ltd., 1995)
Page 119: *Conquest of Mind* by Swami Sivananda (The Divine Life Society, 1962)
Page 157: *Radha: Diary of a Woman's Search* by Swami Sivananda Radha (Timeless Books, 2002)
Page 187: *Bliss Divine* by Swami Sivananda (Divine Life Society, 1965)
Page 195: *Autobiography of a Yogi* by Paramahansa Yogananda (Self-Realization Fellowship, 1979)
Page 197: Krishna Das from liner notes for CD *Breath of the Heart*
Page 200: "Devavani: Sanskrit, Sacred Literature, and the Study of Life" (American Sanskrit Institute)
Page 201: *Meditation and Mantras* by Swami Vishnu-devananda (International Sivananda Yoga Vedanta Centers, 1978)
Page 203: "On Love in Sanskrit," poem by Kirpal Gordon—for more on the work of Kirpal Gordon, visit www.kirpalg.com
Page 205: *Savitri* by Sri Aurobindo (Sri Aurobindo Ashram Press, 1993)

Acknowledgments

I am grateful to the extraordinary men and women in this book, who give so generously of themselves in order that others may do the same. To hear and convey their tales has been a privilege. Thanks also to the posture models—Ghiora Aharoni, Jason Brown, Catherine Ho, and Dana Strong—whose love of yoga graces these pages. I am indebted to Rike Behrendt, June Borup, Hilary Fulton, Eve Harris, and Heidi Hybl for listening; to Jon Cassotta and Michael Hutchison for telling; to Lisa Landphair, for her careful eye in reading the manuscript; to Karen Nuccio and Ms. "Dojo" Metta for keeping me fed; to Sahar F. for digital snaps and to Sebastian Kaufmann, for the emergency laptop; to Emily Seese, for her kind assistance; to Dave at Ananda Ashram for accommodations; and to Elizabeth Juviler, Meher Khambata, Nancy LaNasa, Anne O'Brien, and Elliot Schneider for weighing in. Big-time kudos to premier photographer Andy Ryan, and to Richard Berenson, whose design made the impossible possible. The light within me salutes the light within you.